MEDICAL SURVIVAL

Also by W. Gifford-Jones

HYSTERECTOMY?
ON BEING A WOMAN
THE DOCTOR GAME
WHAT EVERY WOMAN SHOULD KNOW ABOUT
   HYSTERECTOMY

MEDICAL SURVIVAL

W. Gifford-Jones, M.D.

METHUEN

Toronto   New York   London   Sydney   Auckland

Canadian Cataloguing in Publication Data
Gifford-Jones, W.
    Medical survival

ISBN 0-458-99640-8

1. Medicine, Popular. 2. Self-care, Health.
I. Title.

RC81.G54 1985   610   C85-099275-3

Text Design: Patrice Clarkson

Printed and bound in Canada

1 2 3 4   85   89 88 87 86

Contents

Preface

People at parties invariably ask me, "Why do you write a syndicated medical column?" I tell them deadlines have a value. Samuel Johnson remarked, "Nothing sharpens the wit so much as the knowledge you're going to be hanged in the morning." Deadlines also speed up the thinking and help you see the forest as well as the trees. The longer I practice medicine, the more I'm convinced that medical consumers are not getting the right message on how to prevent disease. We can send rockets to Mars, but the art of human communication is very, very difficult.

An economist once remarked, "If you keep going to hell, you'll eventually get there." Today millions of people are on their way to a medical hell. There are two kinds of diseases in the 1980s—the ones we get and the ones we make. During the Korean War post-mortem examinations revealed that 77 percent of dead U.S. soldiers, with an average age of 22, had significant coronary heart disease. One percent of the enemy had it. We are obviously doing something wrong when one person in three will have a heart attack before they're 60. This year 750,000 North Americans will die of heart attacks. It's shocking that 50 percent of the population die of coronary heart disease, and that every 60 seconds a new diabetic is diagnosed in North America.

What has gone wrong? Leonardo da Vinci once made a sage comment: "Nature never breaks her own laws." History has repeatedly shown what happens when you break natural laws. If politicians print too much paper money they ruin the currency. If man continues to pollute the ocean and air he, too, courts ecological disaster. And if you break the natural laws of medicine you court medical disaster.

Some things are obvious. When a man applied for a job at the railroad station, he was asked, "Suppose you saw a train coming from the east at 100 miles an hour. Then you looked west and saw another train coming at 100 mph. The trains were on the same track and just a quarter of a mile apart. What would you do?" The man scratched his head for a moment and replied, "I'd run and get my brother." "Why in the name of heaven would you get your brother at such a crucial time?" he was asked. The man said simply, "Because my brother has never seen a train wreck."

Today millions of North Americans are headed for a massive train wreck. Einstein had a formula that made him famous. I have no delusions about mine. But I'm convinced EP = A + D (extra pounds = atherosclerosis + diabetes). I often tell my patients that obesity is like dancing with a grizzly bear. He may be cute and even play with you for a while. But sooner or later he gives you a lethal whack.

I hope this book will show people how to circumvent garbage diseases. Humans are like computers. If you put garbage into a computer you get garbage back. In order to prevent these problems, you must develop a new psychological and philosophical approach to degenerative disease. You must stop thinking in terms of single diseases like mumps, pneumonia, and coronary heart disease. You must develop a more generalized conception of problems, because it's hard to tell where one degenerative problem ends and another begins. Or what is the cart and what is the horse.

In the 1980s people must also realize there's a very major difference between medicine and religion. Medicine has no benevolent God that forgives past sins and gives you a second chance. Yet day after day I see patients who think they can abuse their bodies for 40 years and still expect doctors to perform miracles.

I also wrote this book because I have much in common with the one-armed economist. Harry S Truman once became irritated during an economic conference in the White House. Suddenly he asked an aide to go out and bring back a one-armed economist. He said he was tired of hearing his advisers say, "But on the other hand. . . ." This book, like the former U.S. president, calls a spade a spade. History will show that there are people in positions of power who are not alerting the public to medical hazards. And there will be a special place in hell reserved for them.

This book will help people to keep an open mind on medical matters but not so open that their brains fall out. For instance, I think the farmers, hens, and cows are getting a raw deal. For hundreds of years the cows didn't cause coronary heart disease. But now the TV tube says butter and eggs are increasing the blood cholesterol and triggering coronary attacks. But blaming the cows for this twentieth-century malady is like blaming the iceberg for sinking the *Titanic*. The real merchandisers of disease today are the multinational companies who pour garbage into unsuspecting consumers.

I didn't forget that variety is the spice of life, so I've covered an array of controversial topics. Should you rob the children's piggy bank to buy vitamin E? How long should career women wait to have their mañana baby? Will a lack of estrogen make menopausal women rob banks? What is the best treatment for common hemorrhoids? How can cancer victims prevent a needless colostomy? Is it possible to obtain better medical care than the rich? How can teenagers prevent catastrophic sporting injuries? How can the experience of the battleship *King George V* save North Americans from a variety of medical problems? What are the ways to avoid needless radiation? And does it make sense to have a scotch and soda after a major operation? Is it safe for women to sit on a public toilet seat? And how the W. Gifford-Jones Living Will can help people die with dignity.

Today we live in an age of electronic marvels that do save lives. But they treat the disease, not the patient. All too often they cause fear in the minds of those stricken with serious disease. The importance of hope is frequently forgotten amid these machines. I trust that this book will provide victims of serious disease with a shot of what's been called psychopenicillin. As Shakespeare said of hope, "Kings it makes gods and meaner creatures kings."

I firmly believe that if you lose your sense of humor, you lose everything. So I've included my famous column on the fractured male organ. I couldn't stop chuckling while writing it. Thousands of readers laughed with me. There was just one exception—the farmer who wrote saying it wasn't very funny. Why? Because it had happened to his prize bull.

The W. Gifford-Jones Foundation

December 20, 1984, will always be etched in my mind. This was the day the W. Gifford-Jones Foundation won a major battle for the alleviation of pain and the right to die with dignity. On this day the Federal Minister of Health in Ottawa announced that heroin would be legalized for medical use in fighting terminal cancer pain.

It has always been my belief that to justify its existence a syndicated medical column must address itself to vital issues that affect the health of this nation. In January 1979 I acted on the best New Year's resolution of my life in the Doctor Game column. I made a plea to the Canadian government to allow physicians to use the world's top painkiller to ease the indescribable agony of terminal cancer victims. This potent narcotic had been available in England for over 80 years. It seemed ludicrous that it was being denied to cancer patients in Canada. Thousands of people agreed that the law had to be changed and wrote letters supporting the medical use of this humanitarian drug.

I thought the evidence in favor of heroin was overwhelming. Heroin is stronger than morphine, more logical for injections, travels to the brain faster, stops the cough reflex in lung cancer patients, relieves apprehension and elevates the mood of dying patients, and kills terminal pain when other drugs fail.

But the road to the legalization of heroin has been a rocky one. Powerful groups have opposed the legalization of this useful and potent narcotic. I have been called a misinformed medical columnist who is spreading false hope. Some have labeled heroin as just a "trendy drug."

The W. Gifford-Jones Foundation was established in 1983 largely as a result of continuing frustration. We had delivered 25,000 letters to the Minister of Health in Ottawa from concerned Canadians. Never before in Canadian history had there been so many letters—three green garbage bags full—delivered to Parliament with such a unanimous verdict about an issue. The Minister of Health agreed to set up a committee to study the medical use of heroin. But she then placed three of the strongest opponents of heroin on this committee. It became apparent that we needed more than letters to fight both the government and other opponents of heroin.

Since that time donations sent to the Foundation have been used to place ads in newspapers. I believe that these ads were largely responsible for bringing about the legalization of heroin.

How did the W. Gifford-Jones Foundation accomplish so much against such opposition? The Foundation is small, doesn't sit on fences, and doesn't like political decisions or committees. We also did our homework. For 29 years politicians and bureaucrats claimed that the World Health Organization had banned the medical use of heroin. The Foundation went to Geneva and found this to be untrue. The Foundation also sent thousands of letters to Ottawa from Canadians supporting the medical use of heroin. We presented several briefs on heroin to the parliamentary committees and met with the Ministers of Health. In the end we won because we had a just cause and the dedicated support of thousands of people who had seen loved ones die in agony. As Victor Hugo once said, "No army can withstand the strength of an idea whose time has come."

But the Gifford-Jones Foundation has not won the war. The Minister of Health also announced that strict protocol would surround the use of this humanitarian painkiller. We believe it is wrong to have political and bureau-cratic controls governing the use of heroin. Any protocol is bad protocol in the management of cancer pain. Heroin should be present in all Canadian hospitals and available to those who die in agony in their home. The politicians do not tell doctors how, when and where to prescribe morphine. The same reasoning should apply to heroin. Good sense dictates that cancer victims want to be treated by their physician, not by their politician. The W. Gifford-Jones Foundation will continue its efforts to fight for the unrestricted medical use of heroin. Physicians cannot stop the agonising pain of cancer in the home when heroin is locked up only in certain hospitals. Doctors would have to be magicians to accomplish that.

1

Lifestyle: Preventive Medicine

Desiderius Erasmus made a simple statement in 1508: "Prevention is better than cure." Shakespeare, not to be outdone, drove home the same point; in the play *Julius Caesar*, Cassius cautions, "The fault, dear Brutus, is not in our stars, but in ourselves." And for years insurance companies have produced convincing statistics that North Americans are killing themselves. But preventive medicine still isn't fashionable. That's why thousands of us will succumb this year to preventable premature deaths. The thoughtful consumer should heed this warning, if not for himself, at least for the sake of his children.

This is a brand new challenge. In the Middle Ages, or even at the birth of our country, it was hard to sell preventive medicine. Why not eat, drink, and be merry? The next day you might die of a fulminating infection. It could result from a simple cut, pneumonia, diphtheria, or a host of other infectious diseases. In those days it would have been a tough task to sell retirement savings plans.

Today's longevity statistics should make us more responsible. But often, without realizing it, we squander away our lives. Some of us have needless coronaries in our 40s. Others set the stage for hypertension and early stroke. Still others may be eating our way towards a preventable cancer of the bowel. Loving parents even steer children into lives of obesity with all the attendant problems.

When most people want to live long and healthy lives, why does this happen? For one thing consumers (even some doctors) forget the prime reason we survive longer nowadays. A lion's share of the credit goes to the flush toilet, proper sewage disposal, clean water, and immunization. Doctors have added the icing to the cake by giving us antibiotics, blood transfusions, anesthesia, and better surgery.

The consumer is misled by repeated stories of medical progress in the cure of other non-infectious diseases. But medicine has really oversold what it can and cannot do. The death rates from cancer, heart trouble, strokes, diabetes, respiratory problems, and cirrhosis have remained about the same for the last 20 years. In fact, in some instances, the death rate has actually increased.

Some of these deaths are acts of God, but an increasing number are self-destructive acts of man. Consumers forget one critical fact: It is your lifestyle that often determines how well and how long you live—not the doctors who cut out cancers, transplant hearts, or prescribe insulin and tranquilizers.

Maybe Yankee Stadium in New York City best portrays what is happening to North Americans. When it was first built in 1900 the seats for the fans were 19 inches wide. When it was renovated in 1976 it lost 9,000 seats. Why? Because the expanding posteriors of Americans meant the width of the seats had to be increased to 22 inches. Fifty million Canadians and Americans are said to be jointly one billion pounds overweight.

Potato-chipping yourself into an early demise is merely one way of committing premature suicide. This chapter will outline some others and, I hope, reinforce the sounding alarm.

More than money is needed to circumvent disease. We've tried that route. The cost is staggering, the results poor. In 1950 Canada and the U.S. spent about $13 billion on health care. This figure soared to around $160 billion in 1977. And just consider what some companies have allocated to employee health programs; last year General Motors spent more money on health care than on steel to build cars.

It's one thing to bankrupt Canada and the U.S. for medical care. It's another matter to do it when the money is used for diseases that should never have happened.

Don't Let Stress Become Distress

When is stress the spice of life? And when does it trigger nervous breakdown, peptic ulcer, hypertension, arthritis, or a coronary attack? Dr. Hans Selye, the internationally famous pioneer in the study of stress and its effect on the body, died in Montreal October 16, 1982. He left many medical legacies to the world. But we should all remember one point in particular—Selye's repeated emphasis that it isn't stress that destroys the body, but rather how you respond to it. Illness strikes only when the reaction to stress becomes distress.

Selye often used this example to drive home his point. "Suppose," he would say, "you meet a helpless drunk. He throws insults at you, but is too inebriated to cause bodily harm. Nothing happens if you ignore him. But if you prepare to fight, you discharge hormones that increase the heart rate and blood pressure, and the nervous system becomes tense."

What can happen from this encounter? The person with coronary heart disease may suffer a fatal attack. Who then is the murderer—the drunk who never laid a hand on you? Or did you commit biological suicide? Selye was convinced that considerable illness is triggered by the choice of the wrong reaction.

Selye began to pinpoint the physiological effect of stress in 1936. He injected extracts of cattle ovaries into rats and noted several changes. Large ulcers appeared in the stomach, the adrenal glands enlarged, and the spleen and lymph nodes decreased in size. He then discovered that other noxious substances produced the same changes. Selye labeled this reaction the General Adaptation Syndrome (GAS).

But how does GAS initiate a bleeding ulcer? Stress first causes an alarm reaction, or as Selye said, "a call to arms" of the body's defensive forces. In some instances stress is so great that death results. But in most cases the body adapts to the stress and creates resistance. Eventually, however, continued stress causes exhaustion, the defence system breaks down, and the gnawing pain of an ulcer begins. Or it could result in tension headache or other stress-related problems.

Avoiding stress is not the answer. As the late Montreal researcher remarked, "Complete freedom from stress is death." There's never been a time in history when humans could avoid all adversity. The secret is to develop a healthy, rather than an unhealthy, response to stress.

How do you foster a healthy reaction to stress? Dr. John H. Howard, Associate Professor of Business Administration at the University of Western Ontario, suggests a way. In his report, "Stress and the Manager," Howard writes, "What seems to differentiate the more successful from the less successful in coping with stress producing situations is their awareness of the stress potential in a situation, their sensitivity to their own reactions and their capacity for alternate responses. Successful coping seems to be a skill in which there is some potential for learning."

Howard says the best technique is to build up resistance by regular sleep, exercise, and sound health habits. Work hard on the job, but blank out job-related problems at home. Use "bitch" sessions for relief, and take a break from stressful situations when possible. The person who builds up physical resistance and who develops a preventive attitude about his health will have the energy to deal with stressful situations rationally and effectively.

Selye's own philosophy can also help us combat tension. He believed that the aim of life is not to work as little as possible. He wrote, "For the full enjoyment of leisure you have to be tired first, as for the full enjoyment of food the best cook is hunger." Those who strive for shorter and shorter work weeks and earlier retirement should take note.

He had other sound advice. Accept the fact that perfection is impossible, but in each category of achievement there is a "best." Be satisfied to strive for that. Try to concentrate on the pleasant aspects of life. And when you encounter a stressful situation, consider first whether it is really worth fighting for. And if you suffer a great defeat, remembering past achievements will defeat depression.

Selye at the end of his life practiced what he preached. He had two artificial hips and at 65 developed a reticulo sarcoma, which is usually fatal. It provided him with the biggest challenge of his life. He could either slide into a death watch or adapt and squeeze as much out of life as possible. He chose the latter and beat his malignancy.

Did Selye just get lucky, or did this adaptation conquer the cancer? We can't answer that question. But researchers have found that when patients have a strong will to live, they make a greater effort and use their immune system against cancer more effectively.

Take a Lesson from the Battleship *King George V*

What can we learn from the British battleship *King George V*? Most people remember it for chasing Germany's mighty *Bismarck*. But along with unforgettable visions of the smoke of battle, Ship Surgeon Captain Peter L. Cleave carries another memory. At the time all 1,500 men aboard the British ship were constipated. Cleave himself suffered from the same affliction. How this happened and how he treated the problem is a key to our own nutritional survival today.

Preventing and curing constipation at sea during wartime is a tough assignment. Fresh fruits and vegetables are scarce commodities. But Cleave abhorred the old routine of handing out laxatives to the crew. So he tried an experiment on himself. For several days he consumed raw unprocessed bran. It worked for him and later for others. And he found another advantage—it also cured many of the sailors' hemorrhoids.

Several years later Cleave made another discovery. In 1946, when he was serving at the Royal Navy Hospital in Chatham, his surgeon-commander was suffering from diverticulitis. It's a disorder in which food becomes trapped in small outpockets of the large bowel, causing inflammation and pain. Captain Cleave relieved his colleague's suffering by using bran.

What eventually happened to Cleave? You might expect he would be made an honorary member of the Royal College of Physicians, maybe a life member of the Naval Academy. And I'm sure many hemorrhoid sufferers would gladly have given him the Nobel prize. Instead, he became known as "the bran man." Often ridicule was heaped on him.

But the critics who laughed should have looked at history books. Hippocrates, the father of medicine, had similar sage advice. In 400 B.C. he recommended that the people of Athens should pass large bulky movements. To ensure this they should eat whole-meal bread, vegetables, and fruits.

During the war with France in the eighteenth century food was scarce. So the British Parliament passed a law to stretch the supply of grain. It meant that 80,000 English soldiers had to eat bread made from unbolted flour. Army doctors noted that their health improved.

History provides other hints. Baron von Steuben was a German officer who trained American soldiers during the Revolutionary War. It may be that he was a trifle biased, but he thought Prussian soldiers were healthier. It was his opinion that the difference was due to their habit of eating unbolted bread.

Sylvester Graham of graham cracker fame similarly had strong views on the medical value of unbolted flour. Moreover, he didn't concentrate his attack just on humans. He repeatedly stressed that cattle were healthier when fed whole grain.

During the 1980s we are also engaged in warfare. It's not as dramatic as fighting the *Bismarck*, but it's much more dangerous than naval warfare. A few thousand sailors may die in the heat of battle. But year after year millions of North Americans are dying because of faulty food habits.

What mistakes do people make? There are several, but a very basic one is ignoring the vital importance of fiber. It's easy to understand why we tossed out fiber over 100 years ago. We thought we were improving on nature when we discarded the hard outer crust of the wheat kernel to make white bread. After all, the crust contains no nutritional value. The body doesn't even digest it. But this was a serious error.

Fiber absorbs water. In the intestines it combines with wastes to form soft, bulky stools. This increased mass turns the bowel into a fast assembly line. The best way to analyze its value is to see what happens when there's a lack of natural fiber.

The stools become hard and small, so the bowel has to muster more strength to push material along. The end result is constipation. This in turn causes hemorrhoids and aggravates varicose veins. It's possible the increased pressure also produces hernias, and there's every reason to suspect it initiates diverticulitis.

But the problem doesn't end with physical straining. A rusty slow bowel is much like a rusty drain pipe. It eventually develops other complications. Look at it this way: if you're careless about throwing out garbage, it piles up and clogs the system, threatening infection and disease. The large bowel is the human disposal dump and is similarly threatened. Scientists believe some leftovers contain cancer-containing compounds. The longer they're left in contact with the bowel, the greater the chance of malignancy. Horse sense suggests that the sooner the body gets rid of waste products the better.

Fiber also helps to fill the stomach with calorie-free substance. This fights obesity, today's number one killer, and thus helps to reduce hypertension, strokes, heart failure, diabetes, and blindness. Sound advice on a mighty battleship ought to be heeded by those of us on land.

Please, Dear Lord, Protect Me from This Goblin

"Please, Lord, protect me from goblins in the night. Grant me the strength never to succumb to the lure of addictive drugs. Shield me from all the over-the-counter nostrums that supposedly benefit my health. Safeguard me from the use of tobacco and excessive use of alcohol. And please, Dear Lord, protect me from the incredible ravages of sugar." This would be my nightly prayer if I were a little boy with the knowledge I have today.

In 1980 the president of a major sugar company remarked that sugar prices could be expected to rise. In the same breath he gave us more bad news. He advised consumers not to hoard as there was plenty of sugar, and that prices would eventually come down.

What a shame! If prices could only rise to $10 a pound, or give the price of gold a run for its money. This one event would prevent untold suffering for tens of thousands of American children.

Last year sugar sales in North America reached 37 billion pounds. That means each person in the United States consumes about 130 pounds of sugar annually. And there's no indication this upward trend will stop.

"Doesn't sugar give you energy?" you ask. "And in an energy-deficient world, isn't energy what we all need?"

But there's a catch to energy derived from sugar. Producers never explain that it contains no vitamins, no minerals, no enzymes, no trace elements, and no fiber. Sugar does not provide any health benefits. It simply loads the body with excessive calories. This makes us fat and exposes us to many diseases.

The list of sugar-related health problems is as long as your arm. The number one disease is tooth decay. Last year the U.S. Navy invited me aboard the *U.S.S. Nimitz*, the largest American nuclear aircraft carrier. The ship's dentists work seven days a week. It's impossible for them to catch up with dental diseases on board, even though the average age of the crew is only 19.

It doesn't have to be this way. For several years dental officers in the British navy carried out a study on Tristan da Cunha, a group of isolated islands in the Atlantic about halfway between Africa and South America. The natives used to subsist mainly on fish and potatoes. In 1938 none of the islanders had decay in their molar teeth. But by 1962 they were all consuming a pound of sugar every week. And their teeth had become rotten.

Boys and girls in North America don't want decaying teeth. And none of them want to die prematurely. But long before they receive their first pair of skates adults set them up for this devastation. The great majority are still in diapers when it begins.

Many American babies are denied natural breast feeding. Instead they are fed infant formulas and baby foods laden with sugar. These produce fat babies, and unfortunately modern society likes bouncing babies. Outwardly they appear healthy, but fat babies almost invariably become obese adults. And today obesity far outranks cancer as the number one killer.

Obesity and an overloaded truck have something in common. A top-heavy vehicle gets flat tires; humans get aching feet. The overworked transmission breaks down in machines and we develop hypertension, atherosclerosis, strokes, and coronaries. Heavy trucks consume more gas and our bodies need additional insulin. This series of interrelated diseases has become an epidemic in our country.

But what an inconsistent society! We all heartily agree it's a criminal offence to push heroin. Yet we encourage the production and consumption of billions of pounds of sugar that will destroy our offspring.

Why do food manufacturers use so much sugar? Because it's cheap and heavy. A cup of flour weighs 100 grams. A cup of sugar is double the weight. So it's more profitable for industry to stuff products with cheap, heavy sugar.

We all consume sugar unknowingly in insidious ways. For instance, we'd think anyone mad who went to the sugar bowl and consumed seven spoonful of sugar several times a day. Yet, daily, Americans swallow a variety of soft drinks that contain this same amount.

Answering my prayer would be a tough job today. We'd need a major uprising like the Boston Tea Party. Until recently I didn't realize how much we're inundated with sugar. Try reading the labels on food packages for a few days; the amount of sucrose and other sugars present in processed food will astound even the skeptic.

My prayer might be possible if we all started by throwing out sugar-coated cereals, commercially baked pies, cakes, cookies, sweetened canned goods, and soft drinks. We should substitute whole wheat for white bread. And put the sugar bowl out with the trash.

The Pancreas, Like a Tired Horse, Can Only Be Whipped So Long

Earthlings should take a long view of themselves. Superior beings on another planet must be aghast at our self-destructiveness. They'd be amazed at the North American custom of inviting preventable disease. They'd watch millions of citizens develop diabetes unnecessarily, primarily because earthlings forget you can only whip a tired horse so long.

My medical professors never stressed the relationship between a worn out horse and diabetes. They taught that diabetes resulted from too much sugar in the blood, that it eventually ended in diabetic coma, that the problem was usually inherited, that insulin controlled it. But they left out the cause of the disease and never taught prevention.

What has a tired horse to do with diabetes? First it's necessary to under-stand how glucose (sugar) is handled by the body. Glucose is the energy of the system. It keeps our hearts pumping, our legs moving, our brain thinking. The average glucose concentration in the blood is about 100 mg. We all develop temporary diabetes after a meal. At this time the amount of glucose rises, and insulin is released from the pancreas to clear the blood of excess sugar, which is stored in the liver as glycogen. When the glucose level falls, glycogen is discharged from this organ. A healthy pancreas is necessary to maintain a delicate balance.

Today's pancreas should go on strike, or at least form a union to get a fairer deal. Some North Americans rarely give the pancreas a rest. They're constantly loading their bodies with excess sugar. They begin the day with sugar-coated cereals. Between meals they pour sugar into coffee or consume sugar-laden soft drinks. They munch on candy bars and delight in fancy desserts. Small wonder that the pancreas rebels at such flogging.

Many people naively blame diabetes on heredity. It is true that a recessive gene is responsible in some cases. But can we have 12 million bad genes in North America?

God didn't create millions of diabetics—we did it ourselves. There's ample scientific evidence to back up this statement. Diabetes is virtually unknown in primitive societies like the Canadian Eskimo, American Cherokee, the natives of New Guinea, and other areas. These people never consume refined sugar or refined carbohydrates such as white bread and spaghetti.

What happens when our so-called advanced civilization refines its eating habits? The big problem is that nothing happens for about 20 years. This leaves the impression that our new ways are sound, that life can be good and sweet without liabilities. But then something begins to give. The pancreas becomes crippled by the constant bombardment of sugar.

Diabetes wields a multi-pronged sword of destruction. It lowers the body's resistance, causing boils, fungus infections, and poor healing after surgery. But primarily it triggers premature aging of the arteries, so that some diabetics succumb to early heart attacks and strokes. Others suffer from kidney failure, lose a leg from gangrene, or become blind.

What a tragedy when this outcome can be prevented. We often hear the expression, "What's in a name?" Surely the name itself should give everyone the clue on how to prevent this disease. It's not called "sugar diabetes" without good reason.

North Americans shouldn't wait for the symptoms of diabetes to appear. By the time there's excessive thirst, urinary frequency, hunger, weakness, weight loss, and itching of the skin, the pancreas is exhausted.

I've heard people make foolish remarks about diabetes: "If you get diabetes today you can take pills rather than needles." Anti-diabetic pills do help some patients. But they're not the panacea that we once believed when they were introduced several years ago. For most, diabetes still means taking injections for the rest of their lives.

There's another point to keep in mind. Canadian scientists Sir Frederick Banting and Charles H. Best gave the world insulin. It was a great achievement and keeps millions of diabetics around the globe alive. But insulin isn't a 100 percent cure. The victims of diabetes still suffer from long-standing vascular complications.

A wise person would try to prevent this disease. He would first accept the fact that refined sugar has been proven to be the plague of civilized man. He'd make dramatic moves to limit household consumption of the culprit. He'd maintain normal weight, keep physically active, and add more fiber to his diet. All these precautions give the pancreas a rest and save it from developing the tired horse syndrome.

There is no doubt that a major epidemic of diabetes is maiming and killing North Americans. There may be a special place in hell for health officials and the presidents of corporations whose company products are fueling the disease. And for others in positions of power who are sitting on their hands and doing nothing to protect the children of this fast-food age. It is the most flagrant lapse of responsibility in the history of medicine.

During talks with public health associations I've repeatedly asked these questions: What would you do if every 60 seconds there was a new case of polio, diphtheria, or smallpox in North America? If you knew large companies' irresponsibility was contributing to the epidemic, and incidentally making a profit for this misfortune? I think there would be a dozen Royal Commissions and Senate Committees appointed to investigate the problem. And it would make headlines in every newspaper in the world.

Yet every 60 seconds there is a new case of diabetes diagnosed in North America. This year another 450,000 people will develop the disease. Between 1965 and 1973 diabetes increased 51 percent in the U.S. Now about 5 percent of the population are brought to their knees by this disorder.

There's a major difference in this epidemic. Years ago if you developed smallpox it killed you. Unlike infectious disease, diabetes triggers a variety of lethal problems. It causes premature hardening of the arteries (atherosclerosis). This in turn sets the stage for hypertension, strokes, heart and kidney failure, gangrene of the extremities, and blindness. Ten percent of blindness today is due to this disease.

Governmental inconsistency about diabetes is mind-boggling. Isn't it ludicrous that government protects us from dirty restaurants, tuberculosis, and measles; that they force us to wear seat belts; that they are concerned about the amount of fat in our diet; that they ban or censor movies to safeguard our morals. Yet they are seemingly unconcerned that a new diabetic is diagnosed every minute. What would happen if a new case of Legionnaire's Disease occurred every 60 seconds?

There's another absurd inconsistency. We're told to beware of the cholesterol in eggs and switch to polyunsaturate margarine. But this is like blaming the iceberg for sinking the *Titanic*. Hens and cows aren't the culprits. It's lifestyle that causes degenerative diseases. But have you ever heard health officials criticize the soft drink manufacturers who pour eight teaspoonsful of sugar into a 10-ounce soft drink? Or the presidents of packaged food companies whose products are laden with hidden sugar? Or the sugar industry? Multinational companies are powerful. It's easier to blame the farmer.

Hens and cows are not creating this avalanche of diabetes. History proves that point. Diabetes was less frequent a few decades ago and was usually due to a defective gene. Now it's 90 percent due to nutritional gluttony.

Canadians used to eat more ham and eggs, raw fruits, and vegetables which provide the body with natural foods and fiber. Today a massive switch has taken place to processed foods loaded with sugar and salt. Diabetes is the result.

Is it possible to stem this epidemic? My crystal ball has never been more pessimistic. I forecast that an increasing number of North Americans will develop the disease. After all how can you combat anything if you're not aware of its danger?

Consider how difficult it is to find a diet drink in most public places. It's a rare possibility in the best restaurants, bars, or on planes. Not in fast food outlets. Or even at social functions of the Canadian Association of Public Health.

It's unlikely that families will bypass sugar-loaded cereals that are pushed by the powerful TV tube, or get rid of Danish pastries, fancy desserts, or other processed foods. Most people won't even switch from white to brown bread or leave the sugar bowl off the table. The sugar industry doesn't have to worry.

A hell-and-thunder evangelical sermon should defend hens and cows but warn North Americans to beware of presidents of corporations whose only interest is the balance sheet. They are the merchandisers of one of today's prevalent diseases. Others should share that responsibility. High on the list is the Canadian Public Health Association. Its mandate is the publication of information and warnings in the prevention of disease. Surely someone in that organization knows that infectious epidemics are past history. And that part of its role today is to alert the consumer to the hazards of self-inflicted diabetes and other degenerative disease. A failure to do so should guarantee that place in hell.

Rare Steaks, Cats, and Toxoplasmosis

"One of these days you're going to regret it," Mrs. G-J often remarks. Not because I've invested in some fly-by-night operation or kicked the neighbor's temperamental police dog. The remark is prompted by a frequent request of mine in restaurants—that I wanted a rare, rare steak. So far my luck hasn't run out. But how "blue" can steaks be before they cause trouble? And can cats trigger needless surgery?

Why hasn't the consumer been informed of this danger? After all, cigarette packages must now alert us that smoking is hazardous to health. Soft drinks similarly caution that saccharin has caused cancer in laboratory animals. Surely supermarkets and restaurants should issue a comparable warning about blue steaks.

Even my favorite restaurant isn't concerned about my well-being. Maybe I don't leave a sufficient tip. But none of the waitresses ever say to me, "You dummy, didn't you take parasitology in medical school? Don't you realize that rare steaks can cause toxoplasmosis? We value your patronage. Please change your order to medium so you can return next year."

A well-informed waitress could present a good case for altering the order. She would tell me not to be fooled by the word "toxoplasmosis." It sounds like a rare tropical disease, one you'd only catch in southeast Asia. She would relate an incredible fact: One-third of the adult population of North America has been infected at one time with this parasite. It isn't an exotic bug and toxoplasmosis can produce a variety of symptoms. Since it mimics other diseases, doctors often miss the diagnosis. For example, it frequently produces enlarged glands, and infectious mononucleosis is suspected first.

Why isn't this common infection a household word? There's a good reason. Patients who develop measles, chicken-pox, and mumps know that something is wrong. The majority of people who contact toxoplasmosis are unaware of the infection, or believe the symptoms are due to a minor problem. It's only by checking the blood for antibodies that a doctor can detect previous infections.

A knowledgeable waitress would say that not everyone is that lucky. One survey showed that 90 percent of patients with toxoplasmosis had enlarged glands in the neck; 40 percent complained of fatigue and general malaise; 37 percent suffered from fever; 32 percent had an enlarged spleen and liver; and 11 percent noticed a rash.

Toxoplasmosis can occasionally cause serious complications. For example, the parasite can attack the liver, lungs, heart, and central nervous system. In children it can cause recurrent convulsions and impaired vision and retard mental development. X-rays of the skull may demonstrate small, irregular areas of calcification.

Dr. Kevin Lake, Assistant Professor of Medicine at the University of Southern California, reported on three interesting cases of toxoplasmosis in the 1979 January issue of *Postgraduate Medicine*. He proved that sometimes doctors need the help of an intelligent waitress to make an accurate diagnosis. Even though the disease was discovered 40 years ago, many physicians are still not thinking toxoplasmosis.

One patient was taken to surgery for removal of an enlarged gland in the neck. The doctor worried it might be due to cancer. Pathological examination showed toxoplasmosis. The second patient was thought to have tuberculosis and sent to a sanatorium. An oral surgeon missed the true cause of the neck pain in the third patient; once again the enlarged gland was excised, only to confirm the presence of this parasitic infection. But neither the surgery nor the TB treatment was required. A blood test could have pinpointed the problem.

How can you circumvent this common infection? Take the advice of a sympathetic waitress and don't order rare steaks or eat raw meat. You should also consider tossing out the cat. The three patients of Dr. Lake's study had cats in their homes. It's known that they sometimes excrete the toxoplasmosis cysts in their stools.

Be patient if this disease is diagnosed. Luckily the glands do not develop an abscess, but they may remain enlarged for over a year. Uncomplicated toxoplasmosis does not require treatment. But severe cases need pyrimethamine and sulfa. The antibiotic clindamycin has also given good results.

Have I changed my order yet? Preventive medicine dictates that I should have devoured my last blue steak long ago. It's a tough decision. But it would put an end to complaints when steaks are delivered medium rare. And my wife would never be able to say, "I told you so."

Laugh at T.V. Commercials and Save Your Kidneys

What will happen if North Americans allow the TV tube to become their doctor? Today pharmaceutical companies are selling hazardous medical nonsense on TV. They're urging the public, young and old, to take extra-strength painkillers for everyday use. But they never mention the terrifying complications of this habit for human kidneys. Consumers should laugh dangerous commercials off the TV screen, and medical associations should mount a massive protest against such unconscionable advertising.

They might emphasize a major discrepancy. Physicians are required to caution patients of possible complications during medical treatment. But TV and radio commercials never warn the public that painkillers can cause severe kidney damage.

No mention is made of the Australian disaster. Statistics show the Aussies to be the greatest pill poppers in the world. Now many are paying a terrible price for their folly; 25 percent of patients on renal dialysis machines in Australia are there for one reason. Painkillers damaged their kidneys.

Renal failure in the past was usually due to generalized disease. For example, diabetes often accelerates atherosclerosis, which gradually destroys kidney function. It's still a major health problem. But in 1953 Drs. Spuhler and Zollinger made a startling discovery. They observed that many middle-aged women were developing renal failure, yet these patients didn't have an underlying medical disease. There was just one clue. They had all consumed excessive amounts of painkillers.

It was initially believed that phenacetin was the culprit. This drug was removed from all products in Australia in 1967. Canada followed suit in 1971. It's still available in parts of the U.S. without a prescription. But taking phenacetin off the market in Australia didn't stop kidney damage. It left doctors with one conclusion. Any common painkiller taken in excess is bad for kidneys.

How many painkillers does the average person consume? We know that North Americans gulped down several thousand tons in 1979. But individual consumption is hard to calculate. Like alcohol consumption, it is underestimated by most people. The wily Swiss dreamed up a clever scheme to evaluate usage. They refused to believe the answers of female factory workers, so each day they searched company garbage cans for empty wrappers. Their survey concluded that 30 percent of working women took more than five tablets a day.

How many 300 mg tablets are needed to produce renal damage? Dr. Priscilla Kincaid-Smith, an authority on kidney disease, noted that Australians on dialysis machines have taken painkillers for three or more years. Extra-strength tablets contain 500 mg and the latest advertised on TV contain 800 mg. Taking two tablets of the strongest dosages every four hours adds up to 9,600 mg. Doctors know that 20,000 mg can be a fatal dose.

Can you protect yourself and your family from the perils of over-the-counter painkillers? First ask yourself what you would do if you were an advertiser with a captive TV audience and a huge budget to hire professionals. As well as a gullible public who wants to believe that Aspirin, Entrophen, Anacin, and Instantine are all different when they all contain acetylsalicylic acid. Today's naive consumer even accepts the theory that one brand is better than another because it dissolves a few seconds faster.

Business people don't moralize when the marketplace offers such a profit-able return. It's much easier to retort, "You can't be your brother's keeper. The nation is full of assorted pains and people seek help." Currently there's only one response to this. Decline that kind of help.

Don't let TV ads insult your intelligence. Who cares how fast a painkiller dissolves? Never purchase a product just because it has extra strength. The greater the potency, the more the risk of renal damage. Don't buy painkillers in bottles of 500 unless you have a chronic arthritic problem. The larger bottle and the ability to purchase it anywhere is a hazardous trend. It gives the impression that painkillers are like peppermint candy.

The Canadian and American Medical Associations should inform their governments of their concern. But consumers should help themselves by making it a national pastime to laugh at pill-pushing TV commercials. A big laugh would save some small kidneys.

"Bingo Brain" Syndrome

Do many people suffer from the bingo brain syndrome? Probably more than doctors realize. I'm sure many physicians have never heard of this malady. And equally sure that bingo brain syndrome is a product of more than just bingo temples.

Dr. W. C. Watson, a staff member of the Victoria Hospital, London, Ontario, aroused my curiosity about this disease in a recent issue of the Canadian Medical Association *Journal*. He reported that a 69-year-old woman was admitted to hospital because of chest pain and mental confusion. She was not intoxicated. Her son commented that his mother had suffered from mild transient confusion in recent months. And that she smoked up to two packs of cigarettes a day.

After three days the patient became quite lucid. Dr. Watson then discovered that his patient was an ardent bingo player three nights a week. By coincidence he himself had recently attended a bingo hall to help raise money for a charitable organization. He stated, "I had never been in such a smoke-filled, polluted, acrid atmosphere in my life. Of the 310 players 304 were smoking. By the end of the evening I was fatigued and had a headache." His conclusion? His patient had recurrent carbon monoxide poisoning from playing bingo!

This is not an isolated case. Dr. Chris J. Kachulis is a specialist in internal medicine in Los Gatos, California. He reported in *Postgraduate Medicine* the case of a 52-year-old woman suffering from irritability and frequent fatigue. In addition she was depressed and complained of inability to breathe deeply. What the doctor found in her blood should shock all smokers. We know that automobile exhaust produces carbon monoxide, a poisonous gas. But so do cigarettes. And when carbon monoxide is inhaled, oxygen is forced out of red blood cells, forming carboxyhemoglobin. As the amount of carbon monoxide increases, these cells become starved for oxygen. The normal carboxyhemoglobin level (CHL) is about 1.5 percent. This patient's level was 9 percent although she was a non-smoker.

Why so high? Dr. Kachulis eventually discovered that her husband smoked two to three packs of cigarettes a day. And she sat with him for hours each day in a small, poorly ventilated room. Her husband, confronted with the facts, refused to stop smoking.

Two years later the patient was admitted to hospital. This time she had suffered a grand mal epileptic seizure. Her previous symptoms continued unabated. Now her CHL was 13 percent. During the two-week hospital stay it fell to 2 percent. Her husband, having witnessed the attack, began to smoke in the garage, and 20 months later she had suffered no further seizures.

Is this bingo brain syndrome common? We don't know yet. No researcher has invaded bingo temples with blood-collecting apparatus and gas detectors to find out. But common sense suggests that it must be a frequent occurrence. Studies have shown that CHLs above 10 percent cause lethargy, irritability, headache, blurred vision, slower reaction, and a decreased ability to concentrate. Currently we don't know if high CHL causes an epileptic attack. Yet levels above 25 to 30 percent can be fatal.

At what level is carbon monoxide in the air hazardous? Federal Air Quality Standards state 9 parts per million (ppm). In industry the level should not exceed 50 ppm.

Researchers found that seven cigarettes an hour smoked in a ventilated room produced levels of 20 ppm. But the person seated next to the smoker might inhale 90 ppm. This level was also reached in an enclosed car after 10 cigarettes. And the carbon monoxide level for both non-smokers and smokers doubled within the first hour. Then doubled again during the second hour.

No one disputes that many car accidents are due to drunken drivers, but who questions the level of CHL? Unlike oxygen, CHL remains in the blood for four hours. And it's been proven that drivers who've inhaled high levels of the pollutant cannot distinguish relative brightness, lose some ability to judge time intervals, and have a slower response to taillights. They also show impaired performance on some psychomotor tests.

Today few rational people would disagree that puffing on cigarettes or pipes has a marked effect on health. Now there's increasing evidence that second-hand smoke is an equal hazard.

This shouldn't come as a great shock. We know that smoking during pregnancy is harmful to a fetus. We know that the children of smoking parents have more respiratory infections. We know that animals exposed to 50 to 100 ppm of carbon monoxide suffer damage to heart and brain.

What can non-smokers do to protect themselves? They should think twice before they play bingo! They should also become more vocal. None of us intentionally inhale carbon monoxide from a car's exhaust. So why should we subject ourselves passively to the second-hand smoke of friends and associates? Particularly when they don't give a thought to us.

Does Medicine Have a Benevolent God?

Unlike religion, medicine has no benevolent God. It is normally an unforgiving science that never pardons past medical sins. For example, I've reported before that patients with advanced atherosclerosis caused by years of a careless lifestyle could not repair damaged arteries. But recent research suggests there is hope for medical sinners.

World War II provided the first clue. The inhabitants of occupied countries suffered from severe food shortages, particularly a marked reduction in the intake of fatty foods such as meat and dairy products. But these countries also had a decrease in the amount of atherosclerosis and deaths from heart attacks. What happened after the war? A generation later Norway, on a fat-laden peacetime diet, had one of the highest rates of coronary heart disease in the world.

Further evidence surfaced during the Korean War. Scientists were shocked to discover that 77 percent of U.S. soldiers killed, whose average age was 22, had coronary arteries narrowed by atherosclerosis. Young Koreans and Vietnamese showed no such damage. North Americans were obviously doing something wrong. But there were no scientific experiments to prove that diet could trigger atherosclerosis. Only a nagging suspicion.

Nikolai N. Antischkow made a first attempt to prove this theory in 1913. He fed rabbits a diet loaded with cholesterol-rich foods, producing atheromatous plaques in their arteries. But there was a conspicuous loophole in this study. Rabbits are vegetarians who normally never develop hardening of arteries. The experiment was poorly designed in feeding rabbits something they normally would not eat, and also in such large quantities.

Pathologists at the University of Iowa carried these studies a step further using Rhesus monkeys. These animals have a normal cholesterol level of 140. For 14 months scientists fed them a cholesterol-rich diet, and their cholesterol level jumped to 700. Autopsy showed their main coronary arteries narrowed 60 percent by atherosclerosis.

Could this trend be reversed? To find out, researchers placed a second group of monkeys on the same diet for 17 months. Then for 40 months they were switched back to a normal diet. Autopsy revealed these monkeys sustained two-thirds fewer atheromatous plaques than the first group.

But what about humans? Dr. David Blankenhorn at the University of Southern California has used both diet and drugs to lower high fat levels in patients who exhibit atheromatous plaques in their leg arteries. X-rays of the vessels 14 months later showed a decrease in the size of these plaques. In another study Dr. David T. Nash of the State University of New York studied coronary arteries also narrowed by fatty deposits. By using drugs to lower blood fats, he halted the progression of the obstruction. He also believes he caused a regression in atherosclerosis in some cases.

Dr. S.L. Wilens reports another interesting study in the *American Journal of Pathology*. He performed autopsies on patients who had lost 10 to 100 pounds during the 12-month period prior to their deaths. He found less atherosclerosis in those people who had lost the most weight. Post-mortem examinations on 800 patients with malignant disease also strongly suggested that atherosclerosis regressed in patients dying of cancer.

Sidney Howard, the playwright, once remarked that, "Half of knowing what you want is knowing what you must give up before you get it." Here the message is clear. Overconsumption of fatty foods leads to atherosclerosis.

In 1984 we are constantly reminded that heart disease and cancer are the major human killers. I disagree. The big killer is atherosclerosis. Without narrowing of the arteries there would not be 800,000 deaths from heart attacks every year. There would be fewer cases of hypertension, strokes, kidney failure, and diabetic complications—gangrene and blindness.

Now for the first time there is hope for those who want to avoid atherosclerotic complications. But my practice tells me North Americans need more than words to change their complacent lifestyle.

Does Lowering Blood Cholesterol Exchange One Devil for Another?

The continuing reaction to the experiments of Antischkow, the Russian pathologist, would make him roll over in his grave. In 1913 professor Antischkow fed cholesterol to rabbits. His finding of cholesterol deposits in the rabbit aortas triggered a controversy that still rages 70 years later. One argument claims the best way to decrease coronary disease is to reduce dietary fat and cholesterol. Another argues that the benefits of reduced cholesterol have yet to be proven. Are we coming closer to the truth today? Or is it possible that lowering blood cholesterol merely exchanges one devil for another?

Dr. Michael F. Oliver, Duke of Edinburgh professor of cardiology at the University of Edinburgh, has been studying cholesterol for 30 years. Unlike many authorities he doesn't defend either theory with missionary-like zeal. But he blames researchers for confusing doctors, nutritionists, and the laity. He recently stressed in the British medical journal, *The Lancet*, that the paradox of cholesterol should be explained to physicians and patients alike.

What is the paradox? Strong evidence exists that high blood cholesterol is related to the development of atherosclerosis, plugging of the coronary arteries, anginal chest pain, and death from myocardial infarction. But evidence is weak that lowering blood cholesterol does any good once coronary symptoms have occurred.

Dr. Oliver admits it's considered heresy to stress this fact. But most people can't lower their cholesterol level much more than 10 percent by strict diet. If the normal level is about 200 mg and your cholesterol is 300 mg, horse sense tells us that decreasing it to 270 won't have any significant effect on atherosclerosis. But headlines and media exposure have convinced some doctors and patients that the struggle against cholesterol is imperative. And it's made millions of dollars for the manufacturers of polyunsaturated fats.

Here's another paradox. Heredity or a good lifestyle often keeps a patient's cholesterol level under 200 mg. But studies now show that such people have a greater risk of developing large bowel cancer. This only applies to males, however. Other studies implicate a low cholesterol level in cancer of the lung, gallbladder, and liver, and leukemia.

Professor Oliver points out other contradictions. For example, the cholesterol levels of healthy Scottish and Swedish males, aged 40, are identical. Yet the coronary death rate is three times higher in Edinburgh. Do Scots worry more than Swedes, smoke excessively, suffer from more hypertension, gout, or diabetes? Or are they drinking too much of their Scotch?

The professor didn't mention other inconsistencies. The Masai tribe, Eskimos, and Benedictine monks all consume diets high in saturated fats. But heart attacks are rare in these people. Why is it that 80 percent of coronary attack victims have normal cholesterol levels? And why do the Israelis, who eat polyunsaturated fats, have one of the highest rates of heart attack in the western world? Obviously other factors come into play.

But how could a lower cholesterol level cause trouble? Professor Oliver reminds us that cholesterol is a vital substance for normal body metabolism. For instance, it is a major component of the cell wall. Cells will not function normally without an adequate concentration of cholesterol. Equally important, cholesterol is responsible for the normal immune defence system of the body. Could a lack of this defence result in cancer?

Also, the cholesterol ester is a crystalline material which acts partly as a scaffold for other structures in the arterial wall. Oliver postulates that excessive reduction of cholesterol might lead to collapse of the wall, thrombosis, and heart attack. And who knows, queries Oliver, perhaps aging cells need more cholesterol, not less.

There's been so much hyperbole in the news about cholesterol that we seldom hear about another proven fact. It's the lipoproteins that transport cholesterol in the blood. Low-density ones are the dangerous ones. High-density lipoproteins (HDL) prevent cholesterol from being deposited in the arterial wall. For example, rats have a high concentration of HDL. It's hard to give them atherosclerosis even with diets loaded with cholesterol.

The Scottish professor's message is crystal clear. The secret of success is good timing. The smart investor purchases gold and silver before it skyrockets in price. The successful health investor tosses out the garbage food, excess calories, and cigarettes early in life. He makes regular exercise a lifelong habit. He, too, will eventually die. But he won't be at the Pearly Gates at 45. Or at 50, trying desperately to exchange one devil for another.

The Truth About Marijuana

Winston Churchill was right about the use of marijuana. He once remarked that, "Men occasionally stumble on the truth, but most of them pick themselves up and hurry off as if nothing has happened." For years there's been a widespread belief that marijuana is a harmless drug. But over 6,000 scientific studies now show that the use of marijuana has profound effects on the body. Dr. Helen C. Jones, a renowned researcher at the University of California, points this out in her book, *The Marijuana Question.*

Marijuana, unlike alcohol, is fat soluble. This means it isn't quickly metabolized and excreted from the body. A single dose can take weeks to be eliminated. So a regular user of pot is never free of this drug.

Marijuana is deposited in the fatty outer layers of the cell. These membranes must remain healthy in order to provide the cells with nutrient and oxygen. But as the drug gradually accumulates in the wall, the efficiency of the cell breaks down. The brain, lungs, and sex organs are particularly vulnerable.

Dr. A.M.G. Campbell of Bristol University in England studied the brain function of 10 British marijuana smokers who exhibited personality changes. X-rays showed wasting of the brain's tissue and enlargement of the ventricles.

For six months Dr. Robert Heath of Tulane University gave monkeys doses of marijuana similar to those of moderate to heavy users of this drug. The monkeys were taken off marijuana for eight months, then autopsy was performed on their brains. They, too, exhibited wasting of the brain and enlargement of the ventricles.

Other research done by Dr. Ethel Sassenrath at the University of California confirmed these findings. She concluded, "It is wishful thinking to assume these brain effects would be limited to monkey primates and not human primates."

Why should there be any doubt that marijuana smoke affects the lungs? After all, it contains 50 percent more cancer-producing hydrocarbons than tobacco smoke. Dr. Forest Tennant, former chief of Drug Abuse for the U.S.

Army in Europe, studied soldiers who had used marijuana for just a few months. He found precancerous changes in cells taken from the air passages of the lungs. It would have taken from 10 to 20 years for comparable changes to have occurred from smoking cigarettes.

Marijuana also carries a potent punch for the reproductive system. In males its use decreases the sperm count and causes abnormalities in the sperm, sometimes enlargement of the breasts, and a decrease in the amount of male sex hormone produced.

In women users regular monthly ovulation may be stopped, causing irregular bleeding. Dr. Peter Fried at Carleton University in Ottawa has noted that pregnant women smoking marijuana gave birth to babies who showed altered visual responses, marked tremors, and a high-pitched cry similar to the newborn of heroin and methadone addicts.

Marijuana causes great stress on the cardiovascular system. The heart rate can increase to 180 beats a minute. This triggers a major effect on the blood pressure. Researchers are also becoming increasingly suspicious that this drug alters the body's immune system.

Never be misled into thinking that marijuana does not cause physical and mental addiction. Marijuana users often become irritable, unable to sleep, and anxious and suffer loss of appetite when they abruptly stop smoking pot.

Dr. Ronald C. Bloodworth, Director of the Psychiatric Institute in Atlanta, offers a more sobering thought. He says that the continued use of marijuana can cause schizophrenia, severe depression, and acute manic episodes.

Marijuana users face another potential danger. They can never be sure that other drugs, such as cocaine, have not been added to pot. Studies show that 96 percent of cocaine users first tried marijuana.

I don't think these findings should surprise anyone. Most of us know you rarely get something for nothing. How can any reasonable person expect to obtain a temporary pleasure from drugs without suffering after-effects? But Winston, why won't people believe the truth?

You Can Lower Your Biological Age

Lucius Seneca, the Roman philosopher and statesman, remarked, "Life is nothing but a journey to the grave." It's still a true but somber thought 2,000 years later. But today there are effective ways of preventing many of the diseases of the past. And unlike the ancient Romans, we also have the choice of remaining younger. One way to prod people in this direction is by personalized health analysis.

In 1950 Dr. Lewis C. Robbins at Temple University and Harvey Geller conducted the first "health hazard appraisal." Twenty-five people answered questionnaires about their personal living habits and submitted blood and urine samples. This enabled Dr. Robbins to describe to each participant the 10 most likely causes of his or her death over the next year, the chance of dying from these diseases, and what steps would reduce the risk.

Currently there are over 200 universities, medical schools, public health organizations, and private organizations that use some version of Dr. Robbins's health hazard appraisal. But today questionnaires are fed into computers to obtain the necessary data. The health appraisal provides an opportunity to see how your health compares with other people of the same age, sex, and race, and in very specific terms tells you how to decrease the risk of various diseases.

Health hazard appraisal has another positive aspect. We all know that smoking is a major health hazard, that it can spark lung cancer, heart disease, hypertension, and strokes. That too much drinking causes cirrhosis. That obesity creates the right conditions for so many degenerative problems. Yet too many people cling to the naive belief that such troubles always happen to the other person.

But the health hazard appraisal isn't talking about anyone else. Suddenly it strikes the individual, "Hey, this report is talking about me. I'm the one with the risk of a 55-year-old. But I could lower my risk to that of a 48-year-old if I got smart." When the bottom line is you, the impact is 10 times more potent. Filling out a detailed questionnaire also makes a person conscious of all the things they're doing wrong. It comes as a shock to many people how many cocktails and how much candy they consume every week when forced to keep track of these items.

The 10 major causes of death for men between the ages of 50 to 59, in decreasing frequency, are heart disease, lung cancer, stroke, cirrhosis of the liver, cancer of the large bowel, suicide, bronchitis, and emphysema, pneumonia, car accidents, and diabetes.

For women between the ages of 50 to 59 it's heart disease, breast cancer, lung cancer, stroke, cancer of the large bowel, cancer of the ovary, cirrhosis of the liver, diabetes, rheumatic heart disease, and pneumonia.

Lowering your health risk for these diseases is not a complicated problem. For some people it may be the simple act of using a car seat belt. Or examining the breast every month, decreasing the consumption of red meat and processed foods, adding more fiber to the daily menu, taking fruit, mineral water, or decaffeinated coffee during morning breaks rather than sweet rolls, cakes, and coffee, decreasing the number of alcoholic drinks from 14 to 7 a week, tossing the sugar bowl and the salt shaker off the table, getting an annual Pap smear and regular bowel examinations, and walking up stairs instead of using an elevator.

How effective is the health questionnaire in preventing disease? Dr. Robbins says that after one year people can lower their risk age by as much as four to eight years. The average is about 1½ years. But lifestyle changes don't affect all diseases to the same extent. For example, if you stop smoking, the risk of a heart attack drops almost at once, but the risk of lung cancer decreases at a slower rate.

Nor can improved lifestyle guarantee longer life in all cases. But it does improve the odds. And I'm sure that our effective use of today's knowledge of how to avoid the grave for another eight years would impress Lucius Seneca.

A Forceful Hug Can Break a Rib

Two investors decide to withdraw funds from the bank at the same rate every day. The person with less money obviously goes broke first. Today millions of North Americans are similarly going broke. They're gradually losing their bodies' supply of calcium, some faster than others. And this is causing thousands of needless fractures. For some victims even a forceful squeeze will break a rib.

It's been a well-kept secret that women lose 1.5 percent of their bone mass every year. This continual mining of calcium primarily affects the vertebrae and bones of the hip, shoulder, and wrist. Some women lose as much as six inches in height as the vertebrae gradually crumble.

A report from the Mayo Clinic indicates that one in every four post-menopausal women suffer from thinning, brittle bones. That after age 60, 80 to 90 percent of broken hips occur in women. That women are 10 times more likely to break the lower arm. That every year 1.3 million fractures occur in the U.S. due to osteoporosis in patients over 45 years of age. The cost? $3.8 billion.

The 230,000 hip fractures that occur every year in North America present an enormous problem. Twelve to 25 percent of the victims are dead in one year; 25 percent never walk again. The remaining 50 percent walk with great difficulty. The result is social isolation and depression.

It's understandable that people pay so little attention to bones. The human skeleton, unlike muscle tissue, gives the appearance of never changing. But it is being reshaped constantly during a lifetime. Up to age 35 most people form more bone than they lose. Later, the rate of bone absorption increases and less bone is replaced.

What makes a bone snap like a dry twig? A major factor in women is the sudden decrease in the female hormone, estrogen, at menopause. Lack of estrogen causes decreased calcium absorption and an increased loss of calcium through the urine. White women are more susceptible than black women, but this is even true for Bantu women in Africa when they have too many pregnancies, prolonged nursing, and an inadequate diet of calcium. Daughters of affected mothers are also more likely to develop osteoporosis.

Drugs such as cortisone, tranquilizers, and antacids may also retard calcium absorption. Alcohol consumption, too much caffeine, and a high fiber intake are known to cause an increased loss of calcium in the urine.

Osteoporosis, like diabetes, gallstones, and diverticulosis of the large bowel, is largely a disease of affluence and decadence. Western diets have a high protein content that accelerates calcium loss. Extensive surveys have revealed that the average woman consumes less than 500 mg of calcium a day. But she needs 1,000 mg a day before menopause and 1,500 daily afterward.

Lack of exercise is a big contributor to broken bones. Astronauts lose bone mass in a weightless environment. So do bones kept immobile in a plaster cast. Physical stress strengthens the heart and muscles—it's equally good for bones.

The best way to stop the cannibalization of bone tissue is to trust farmers, hens, and cows. Some patients require calcium tablets, but for most it's wiser to get calcium from the grocery store than over the drug counter.

Those who call milk "nature's most nearly perfect food" are close to the truth. Two glasses of milk contain 500 mg of calcium. Six ounces of hard cheese provide another 500 mg. Yoghurt, milk concoctions such as creamy soups, milk puddings, ice cream, milkshakes, sardines, salmon, and almonds are other sources of calcium. Don't forget leafy vegetables. After all, that's where the cow gets her calcium for milk. Persuading children they can't replace milk with soft drinks will enable them to build up bones that last a lifetime.

Multinational companies could also help to fight this crippling disease if they added bone meal to processed meats during manufacture. This would bring the nutritional value of human food up to the level we expect for dog and cat food. In the United Kingdom wheat flour is fortified with calcium carbonate.

An economist once remarked, "If you keep going to hell, you'll eventually get there." Today millions of North Americans are heading towards a medical hell. Osteoporosis, like many other degenerative diseases, is the result of a poor lifestyle. What a tragedy when it could be prevented by walking to the corner store and making milk a lifetime food, and if women wouldn't listen to the prophets of doom who condemn estrogen therapy for the menopause.

2

Vitamins

The Vitamin E Controversy

Scientists should create a test-tube baby programmed to tackle medical problems. They should start with the genes of Perry Mason, then add those of scientists with the intelligence of Einstein. And they shouldn't forget the chromosomes of philosophers with the wisdom of Solomon. Possibly that mixture would possess the right brain to solve the vitamin E controversy. In essence, the question is: Is this vitamin one of the biggest medical and economic hoaxes of the century? Or should we be robbing the children's piggy banks to purchase it at any cost?

Vitamin E is a multi-million dollar business in North America. Its proponents claim it can be used to treat or prevent heart disease, diabetes, skin ulcers, burns, thrombophlebitis, frostbite, and infertility and improve athletic prowess. They also say it's good for menopause, takes the itch out of old scars, and protects the lungs from pollution. And if you happen to have a hunting dog with an ailing heart, a few thousand units for him will have him running again.

Like most doctors I had never delved deeply into the reason for or against vitamin E. But I thought it would be an easy task deciding whether or not to break open the children's piggy bank. It was a major error that cost me untold hours of research. I read several books on the subject. Then I examined some of the 4,000 research papers on vitamin E. I soon encountered the big problem.

Some international researchers give the impression that vitamin E is the latest version of old-fashioned snake oil. It is supposed to help everything, but cures nothing. Other equally prominent scientists don't agree with these skeptics. But both groups are too respectable to shout from the back of a covered wagon peddling remedies. So who do you believe?

First, how did all the controversy begin? Fifty years ago researchers raised a colony of rats whose diet contained all the essential elements except lettuce. They thrived well and mated, but their offspring all died. Adding lettuce or alfalfa to the menu produced normal offspring. The missing substance was found to be vitamin E.

Researchers then fed a diet deficient in vitamin E to several types of animals. Rats developed liver degeneration, and sperm-producing cells in the

23

testicles were destroyed. Calves were felled by heart damage. Chickens contracted crazy chick disease from brain degeneration.

Experimenters then gave rats more vitamin E than was in their normal diet. These rats could run longer on the treadmill. They could also survive in an oxygen-deficient atmosphere that killed other rats. When the scientists then turned to humans, they found that vitamin E increased the life span of lung cells. And red blood cells also resisted air pollutants when given additional E.

No one raised an eyebrow about these findings. Doctors nodded in agreement again in 1967 when vitamin E finally found a disease to treat. Eleven premature infants with hemolytic anemia (a premature destruction of the red blood cells) were diagnosed as having a deficiency of vitamin E. An E supplement cured the problem.

But for the previous 20 years medical heads had been shaking skeptically. Why? Because two doctors, the Shute brothers in London, Ontario, said they didn't care what small doses of E did for the body. The important fact was that large doses of what they called Big E did help heart disease and many other problems.

The Shute brothers said they had cases to prove it. They also publicized their views with angelic fervor. Evan Shute, writing in the Shute Foundation Summary, put it very bluntly. He said, "We didn't make vitamin E so versatile. God did. Ignore its mercy at your peril."

These ecclesiastical pronouncements were labeled unscientific and unfounded by the medical community. Some said the Shutes tried too hard to sell their product. Others passed them off as charlatans and quacks. A few doctors couldn't get the same results with vitamin E. So for years the controversy continued unabated.

One enterprising bar owner is 100 percent in favor of vitamin E. He offers his customers cocktails with a vitamin E capsule in lieu of the traditional cherry or olive. Other people are buying millions of dollars' worth of this vitamin from health food stores and pharmacies. Will large doses of Big E prolong your life or merely help to empty your bank account? It's strictly dependent on who you talk to.

One prestigious publication says there's no convincing evidence that Big E is effective for treating heart disease or any other human disorder. Another equally weighty medical report says the claims for vitamin E are either excessive or false. Why?

There are ample amounts of vitamin E in many foods, particularly vegetable oils. It's also a fat-soluble vitamin that is easily stored in fat tissues. And since it is eliminated slowly from the body, a vitamin E deficiency is practically unheard of in humans.

The other side claims these statements are insufficient. They say that stored rice, corn, and wheat flour lose half their vitamin E in eight days; that frozen and cooked foods end up deficient in E; that the longer a food is stored or the more it is processed, the less vitamin E it contains. So they think many people get insufficient amounts of the vitamin. They also contend that suggested daily amounts have been set far too low. And lastly, they say it's the larger Big E amounts that protect you from heart and other diseases.

But how can vitamin E do so much for so many different problems? The proponents say that the diseases seem unrelated on the surface but do have a common denominator: Injured or old blood vessels that reduce the supply of oxygen to the tissues. Vitamin E increases the circulation, acts as an anti-clotting agent and decreases the amount of oxygen needed by these organs. And by preventing the oxidation of polyunsaturated fats it also helps you live longer.

Researching vitamin E proved to be frustrating and full of contradictions, but also fascinating, because I eventually zeroed in on facts that don't add up.

For instance, some critics argue that Big E has merely a psychological effect on patients. No doubt that does happen to some extent. But what about the rats that survived in a low-oxygen atmosphere that killed other rats? How could you trick these rats into thinking they were not going to die?

Racehorse owners know how to pick a winner and also have a healthy respect for money. Why would they give Big E to their thoroughbreds if the results didn't warrant it? Oats are much cheaper than vitamin E.

You also get an interesting reaction from doctors. They're often embarrassed to admit taking it. Some wouldn't until I said I was on it. (I wasn't at the time.) It was obvious that numerous physicians are sneaking into the closet to swallow the pill; the records of one pharmaceutical company prove that point.

Other positive findings kept creeping into the research. A prominent surgeon reported using Big E in patients who had suffered major injuries. He thought the anti-clotting properties of vitamin E prevented blood clots from forming in the legs. So why wouldn't it do the same thing for the coronary vessels in the heart?

Even some of the skeptics thought Big E could help a condition called intermittent claudication. The clogged blood vessels in the legs are unable to carry sufficient oxygen to the tissues, resulting in severe pain. Vitamin E sometimes increases the blood supply and eases the symptoms. Why wouldn't it do the same thing for patients who suffer from the pain of angina? After all the heart is only a couple of feet away.

We know that there are a considerable number of rogues in the world. But are all the hundreds of international scientists who have good things to say about vitamin E dishonest or incompetent? You have to be a terrible skeptic to put that label on all of them.

Vitamin E has been given to U.S. astronauts to combat space anemia. It was in the diet of the great racehorse Northern Dancer. And when I eventually discovered that Pope Pius XII and Pope John XXIII had been given it, that clinched the deal for me. If they weren't going to take a chance of having a premature demise, why should I? But I'm not going to sneak into the closet. It's right beside the typewriter, and I hope it keeps me hitting the keys for a long time.

Vitamin E: The Other Side of the Story

Dr. Hyman J. Roberts at the Institute for Research in West Palm Beach, Florida says the purported safety of vitamin E deserves careful scrutiny.

Roberts reported in the British journal, *The Lancet*, that there was an association between megadoses of vitamin E and the occurrence of thrombophlebitis. His study lasted 10 years with patients ranging from 25 to 79 years of age. Two of the 79 patients were taking less than 400 units of vitamin E daily. The rest were consuming 800 or more units a day.

Discomfort and tenderness in the legs, with or without swelling, were the most common symptoms. These troubles disappeared after the patients stopped vitamin E. In addition, pulmonary embolism (blood clot in the lungs) was thought to have occurred in 57 percent of these patients.

His conclusion? Vitamin E can encourage blood clots in patients who have underlying cardiovascular, metabolic, or endocrine disease. No one is certain why this happens. Roberts speculates it may be due to an increase in the blood's platelets, the production of abnormal red cells, an increased immune response, or an increase in the amount of cholesterol, triglycerides, and other lipids in the blood.

Albert J. Kligman of Philadelphia, writing in the *Journal of the American Medical Association*, sounds another note of caution. He reports seeing an unusually high prevalence of emotional disorders with dosages of 800 units a day. The most common symptoms include depression, withdrawal, mood swings, and loss of confidence.

Other physicians are convinced that the self-administration of vitamin E can trigger a severe fatigue syndrome. They say that vitamin E toxicity ranks second only to depression as a cause of tiredness in younger patients.

There's more bad news. Dr. Victor Herbert of New York City reported in the *Journal of the American Pharmaceutical Association* that high dosages of vitamin E caused blurred vision. This may be related to the fact that vitamin E antagonizes the action of vitamin A.

Other researchers believe that too much vitamin E results in enlargement of the breasts in both males and females. That it may cause the development of breast tumors. That it has adverse effects on the metabolism of the adrenal, pituitary, and thyroid hormones. That the white blood cells are less effective in combating infection. And that abnormal vaginal bleeding, diarrhea, dizziness, intestinal cramps, and hypoglycemia may be triggered by excessive amounts of vitamin E.

Vitamin E has also been incriminated as a cause of hives, chapping of the lips, and contact dermatitis. Some patients have developed allergic skin lesions after using a deodorant containing vitamin E.

Everyone agrees on this point. Patients with either a damaged heart or hypertension must always take vitamin E under medical supervision. Vitamin E, by improving the tone of the heart muscle, could further increase the blood pressure.

Albert Kligman points out that most patients have no clear idea why they are taking vitamin E. He also believes evidence is mounting that large doses of vitamin E can cause serious side-effects. Formerly he simply made a note on his record about the intake of vitamin E. Now he strongly recommends that patients discontinue this medication. He also leaves us with a sobering thought —that North Americans are not dumb, but they are among the world's greatest suckers.

Vitamins Can Be Lethal

Suppose a young child begins to complain of increasing fatigue, loss of appetite, and then develops kidney failure. Then another child develops extreme irritability, a fever, and pains in the bones. What would be the most likely diagnosis? Fulminating infection of the kidneys? Tuberculosis? A rare bone tumor? An imported Asiatic germ?

Three pediatricians recently reported cases of this kind. They were setting up doctors for a big surprise. The culprit wasn't a strange virus. In one case it was a loving grandmother who owned a health food store. She was gradually killing her grandchild with kindness. The final diagnosis? An overdose of vitamin A! The other case? Vitamin D poisoning.

Vitamin poisoning has also affected several adults. Sooner or later it had to happen. Last year Canadians and Americans consumed about 30 million pounds of vitamins. And some of them made a grievous error. They assumed that if a little is good for you, more must be better. Their symptoms present a doctor with a difficult diagnosis unless he's thinking "hypervitaminosis."

A Polish biochemist, Casmir Funk, started the vitamin craze in 1922, when he isolated a substance from unpolished rice that prevented beriberi. It wasn't too long before researchers linked the lack of vitamin C to scurvy and the deficiency of vitamin D to rickets. These diseases now belong to history books, but North Americans continue to swallow vitamins in alarming quantities.

Some people are vitamaniacs. They're convinced that multivitamins improve general well-being. Others believe that large doses of vitamin C prevent colds or that vitamin E forestalls heart attack. And much of the population is sure that injections of vitamin B_{12} cure nearly everything.

But who really needs vitamins? People who follow a strict diet for medical necessity or a food fad may require a vitamin boost. So do people who obtain most of their calories from alcohol. Poorly fed senior citizens, post-operative patients, and pregnant women are also helped by vitamin supplements. Most people who devour vitamins, however, are suffering from an emotional deficiency, not a vitamin one.

So often it's been shown that too much of a good thing is worse than none at all. For instance, swallowing over 100,000 units a day of vitamin A spells trouble. The eyebrows disappear, the lips become cracked, and the liver increases in size. Weakness, vomiting, and severe headaches also occur.

There's another bear trap in the far north. Hunters may track down a polar bear, kill it and think they've won the contest. But the bear may have the last laugh. Its liver contains massive amounts of vitamin A. Unwary hunters who eat it have been known to develop acute vitamin A poisoning.

Too much vitamin D can also have a disastrous outcome. Some people mistakenly believe that large doses will ease the symptoms of rheumatoid arthritis. Yet taken to excess, it raises the level of calcium in the kidneys. Renal failure may be the final outcome.

What about the safety of vitamin C? It has been heralded by some authorities as the great cold remedy. Yet others argue that too much causes diarrhea and precipitates the formation of kidney stones.

Multivitamins are much like the snake oil peddled by old-time hucksters from covered wagons. They're not needed, but luckily the amounts don't cause any harm.

Consumers should be wary of fads that concentrate on one vitamin. For instance, a recent lay article recommended high doses of vitamin A as a cure for heavy menstrual bleeding. If that failed to work, the author suggested adding some vitamin E. And for a final try you could also throw in some zinc. Always be careful of this type of self-diagnosis and self-medication.

People who eat a balanced diet of meats, cereals, dairy products, citrus fruits, and vegetables generally don't need extra vitamins. Nor should they be fooled by the word "vitamin." It sounds essential to one's health and far removed from causing injury, but in fact it's a drug that has to be handled with care. Remember that an overdose of vitamins can cause damage to organs before major symptoms appear.

What's Good for the Gorilla May Be Good for Humans

Do today's humans have anything in common with gorillas? Not much, it seems. Gorillas don't poison their environment. They never wage devastating wars or annihilate thousands of defenceless offspring with chemical warfare and starvation. So my apologies to this proud species for linking them in a small way with us. But in the process of evolution we both developed a genetic defect; neither of us can manufacture vitamin C in the liver. Practically all other animals except the guinea pig and the Indian fruit bat have the ability to do so. This metabolic defect may have far-reaching implications for humans.

Researching gorillas was a refreshing and enlightening change. It also left me with a perplexing thought. Are gorillas getting a better deal than humans?

Curators told me repeatedly that the use of vitamin C is routine and "rarely if ever questioned" for gorillas. They say it's been a long-standing practice to utilize C to counteract disease in these captive animals.

G.H. Bourne in 1949 showed that gorillas in the wild receive about 5,000 mg of vitamin C every day from eating fresh vegetation. Dr. Linus Pauling, the Nobel Prizewinner, speaking to biomedical students at the University of Pennsylvania, also revealed a startling fact. He said that goats the size of a man manufacture 13,000 mg of C in the liver day after day. Yet medical authorities insist that humans need a mere 45 mg a day. Should there be such a discrepancy between humans and gorillas?

No one today argues that a severe lack of vitamin C causes scurvy. This deficiency disease produces widespread hemorrhage into tissue, bleeding gums, and eventual death. Jacques Cartier's sailors in 1535 were spared this problem by the North American Indians, who taught them to make a brew from the tip of the spruce tree branch. Later on Dr. James Lind, a naval surgeon, used lime juice to prevent scurvy in British sailors.

But how much vitamin C is required to maintain good health? As in many medical issues, there are two sides to the story. But there is very convincing evidence that North Americans would enjoy better health if they were fed by zookeepers.

Indications are that vitamin C helps to prevent heart attacks and strokes by combating atherosclerosis (hardening of the arteries). Several reports show that heart attacks are less likely in those who consume high levels of this vitamin. How vitamin C protects humans against these arterial diseases is still debatable. But we do know that C is needed to manufacture collagen, which cements cells together. This may result in stronger arteries that are more able to stand the wear and tear of time. It's also an established fact that C has great healing powers. It's always given to patients with extensive burns. So if arterial injury occurs it is more quickly repaired. Moreover, vitamin C aids in controlling the level of blood cholesterol.

Vitamin C combats infection. The body's white blood corpuscles must contain adequate amounts of C to enable them to fight bacteria. In 1935 Dr. C.W. Jungsblut of Columbia University discovered that vitamin C protected monkeys from paralysis by the polio virus. Another important finding occurred in Japan. Patients who receive blood transfusion occasionally develop serum hepatitis. Dr. A. Murata found that patients who were given 2,000 mg of vitamin C avoided this viral disease.

A continuing debate concerns vitamin C and the common cold. Dr. Linus Pauling advocates taking extra C regularly to prevent colds and the consumption of large amounts when a cold strikes. Its been proven that colds and physical exertion increase our needs for C. Possibly that's why Canadian Army troops in Arctic exercises and students in a Swiss ski school are given C. Other studies by T.W. Anderson, Professor of Epidemiology at the University of Toronto, have failed to confirm Dr. Pauling's work. But even if C doesn't aid this common annoyance, it has a vital role to play. For example, experiments are trying to determine if it helps to prevent cancer of the large bowel.

Zookeepers speculate that gorillas receiving vitamin C survive better in our increasingly polluted world. Vitamin C counteracts poisons such as arsenic, nitrates, coal-tar dyes, and many industrial pollutants. But gorillas are exposed to fewer pollutants than humans. They don't sit in traffic jams for hours breathing carbon monoxide fumes. They are not invited to the smoke-filled meeting room for a three-martini luncheon. Nor do they inhale the smoke of a daily pack of cigarettes.

Who said that humans were the advanced species?

Vitamin C and "Aging Arthritis"

I take 500 mg of vitamin C every morning. Why? Some of my colleagues claim that it helps to prevent the common cold. Others contend it decreases the possibility of large bowel cancer. But there's also evidence that vitamin C works to keep cartilage healthy and slows down the onset of osteoarthritis. And I'm thinking I may play tennis longer with the addition of vitamin C than without.

Aging arthritis is a disease of the large joints, involving the cartilage that covers the ends of bones. If one lives long enough, it's impossible to escape this trouble. Virtually everyone over 60 years of age has x-ray evidence of this problem, one of wear and tear. Today it's estimated that 35 million North Americans suffer from arthritis of the large joints, and that 1 in 10 patients who visit a doctor complain of this disorder.

Young cartilage is smooth, tough, and glistening. But with the passage of time it becomes softer and less elastic from constant use. Eventually, in some patients, it becomes so thin that bone ends rub against each other. Continual grating causes opposing surfaces to form rough spurs. The resultant irritation of nerves causes chronic pain and swelling.

Can we fight the development of aging arthritis? Studies indicate that the body is initially able to combat early arthritic changes. But without assistance it gradually loses the battle.

In 1947, Dr. G.H. Bourne, a British researcher, gave guinea pigs varying amounts of vitamin C. He then made small cuts in their skin. The resulting scars were four times stronger when they received 2 mg of C a day rather than 0.25 mg. Dr. J.A. Wolfer confirmed these findings in humans the next year.

Then in 1961 Dr. B.E. Englemark and F.G. Evans made a significant discovery. They showed that the quality of collagen, the primary substance of cartilage, was dependent on the amount of protein and vitamin C available. A lack of vitamin C caused a general weakening of the cartilage and the joints became tender.

Dr. Linus Pauling, the Nobel Prizewinner, has preached the value of vitamin C for years. He's convinced that vitamin C is the kingpin of the body's protective mechanism and that because of a faulty diet humans consume inadequate amounts of C.

The U.S. Department of Health confirmed this fact in 1972. It conducted a survey of 10,126 people in different geographical locations of the country. Fifty percent of these people consumed less than 57 mg of C a day, and 33 percent less than the recommended 45 mg a day.

Dr. James Greenwood is professor of neurosurgery at Baylor University in Texas. He reported in 1980 that 500 mg of C help to maintain the strength of spinal intervertebral discs. He believed that more patients with disc problems could avoid surgery by taking large amounts of C. And he noted that when his patients stopped taking vitamin C after months or years, their symptoms recurred. Discomfort vanished when they started back on C again.

Not all physicians are so sure about the value of vitamin C. Some vitamins are fat soluble and excess amounts are stored in the body. Vitamin C, conversely, is water soluble, and what isn't needed is quickly excreted in urine. In essence, they say, those of us who spend money on C have the most expensive urine in the country.

How much vitamin C is needed? There's no magic figure. Dr. Linus Pauling says that several thousand milligrams a day are required. Possibly he's right if the body is fighting a severe infection; we know that infection rapidly uses up vitamin C. But for those in good health, 500 mg a day seems to be an adequate dose.

Remember that vitamin C won't work miracles. It's unable to ease the pressure on the sciatic nerve from a severely ruptured intervertebral disc, or change badly deformed joints into normal ones. Vitamin C is for prevention. I think it's credible that it helps retard the development of aging arthritis in the wrists of pneumatic drill operators, that it aids the prevention of cartilage breakdown in the knees of football players, and possibly also in the ankles of ballet dancers. And I sincerely hope it keeps me on the tennis court long after the skeptics are in rocking chairs.

Trace Elements

A small hole will eventually sink a big ship. Similarly the gradual accumulation of trace elements in the body can cause hypertension, memory loss, nervous disorders, and sexual impotence. What are these harmful micronutrients? And can the good ones help medical consumers circumvent such potential health problems?

The earth is made up of over 90 elements. But only 26 are essential to health. Eleven, such as calcium, potassium, and phosphorus, are present in relatively large amounts in our food. The other 15 are trace elements, and there is a delicate balance among them.

Today, in an increasingly contaminated world, we should start thinking, "copper." It's essential to health, but all we need every day is about 2 mg. Most people ingest from 3 to 5 mg.

The largest source of copper comes from drinking water. Two things have happened since we replaced zinc-lined galvanized pipes with copper plumbing: We get too much copper and not enough zinc. Copper is also present in a variety of foods such as liver, oysters, lobster, nuts, chocolate, soybeans, and molasses. A biological antagonism exists between copper and zinc; the more we have of one, the less we have of the other. The ideal ratio is to have 14 times as much zinc as copper.

Dr. Carl C. Pfeiffer, a U.S. expert on trace metals, has shown that many hypertensive patients have high levels of copper and low amounts of zinc. Treating these patients with vitamin C plus zinc can result in a decrease in the blood pressure.

Aluminum, unlike copper, is not needed by the body. Most North Americans believe its use is limited to foodwrap, TV dinner plates, and pots and pans. But aluminum is also present in toothpaste, deodorants, cosmetics, table salt, and food additives. Scientists are still not certain how this micronutrient functions in the human body. But the presence of too much aluminum has been suspected as a cause of loss of memory (Alzheimer's disease).

Stomach antacids that contain aluminum hydroxide gel can also reduce the amount of phosphate in the blood. This can aggravate osteoporosis, a thinning of the bones seen in older people, intensify an existing anemia, and exert a toxic effect on the heart.

Bismuth, another non-essential trace element, needs careful monitoring. Bismuth is present in over-the-counter remedies for stomach upsets and diarrhea. It was noted in 1972 that Australians who consumed bismuth compounds for regulation of bowel movements developed the "acute brain syndrome." They experienced disturbances in vision and hearing, loss of memory, and had trouble moving their limbs.

Bismuth salts taken for a few weeks can help to heal peptic ulcers. But their prolonged use results in poisoning. More cases of bismuth poisoning would be detected if doctors started to look for this problem.

The good trace elements can help to fight these troubles. For instance, molybdenum, manganese, and zinc help to rid the body of excess copper. But some North Americans are deficient in these micronutrients. "Fast foods" lose their molybdenum in preparation. Processed white flour loses it with the loss of bran, and the refining of white sugar loses it to molasses. Scientists suspect that a lack of molybdenum is related to dental caries, cancer of the foodpipe (esophagus), and a loss of sexual potency in older males.

Luckily there's an easy way for aging males and others to sidestep these problems. Molybdenum and manganese can be obtained by consuming wholegrain cereals, oatmeal, nuts, seeds, and navy beans. There is also more manganese in tea than in coffee.

Today medical consumers have been programmed to rush to the drugstore for every minor ache and pain. But remember you rarely get something for nothing. Buffered aspirin contains aluminum, and older patients should stay away from the aluminum in many antacid preparations. Pepto Bismol also has bismuth. We get enough of such non-essential trace elements in our food, water, and air without adding to them.

3

Teeth

The Gifford-Jones Dental Pack: To Keep Your Teeth a Lifetime

Why are people so careless about their teeth? Every week I see dental cripples in my office, young patients with complete dentures, otherwise attractive women who refuse to smile because of large, gaping holes in their mouths. Some even suffer from poor nutrition due to a near-toothless mouth. But it doesn't have to happen that way. The Gifford-Jones Dental Pack would prevent the nation's number one disease. No one would every say to you, "The teeth are OK but the diseased gums have to come out." Nor would you be led astray by antiquated and unrealistic TV commercials expounding the virtues of pearly white teeth.

Miguel de Cervantes realized the importance of sound teeth 400 years ago. He wrote, "For I would have you know, Sancho, that a mouth without molars is like a mill without a stone, and a tooth is more precious than a diamond." Yet, today most people still don't appreciate the importance of that message. Tooth decay affects 96 percent of the population. Two out of five Canadians over 19 have lost teeth, and vast numbers of the population eventually succumb to gum disease.

Why have we made so little progress in combating this common problem? It hasn't helped having the three largest soap companies in the world directing most of the dental care. For years, they've been misleading people that they can brush their way to a big, white smile with a little dab of their particular product. This may work temporarily. But brushing solves only half of the problem. Toothpaste companies never suggest that their products are useless in the face of existing gum disease or that they don't clean between the teeth.

I've never seen a toothpaste commercial that instructed children or adults in complete dental hygiene. The old *Amos and Andy* radio shows advised seeing a dentist twice a year. TV commercials now expound the value of fluoride. Or that their new flavor and stripes will ensure a fresh mouth, maybe even a goodnight kiss. But they've never sold this country a reliable total package.

I'd like the Gifford-Jones Dental Pack to give them competition. It's not a new idea. Professor Givanni of Padua, Italy, said in the fifteenth century, "If all particles of food were removed from between the teeth after each meal and the mouth cleansed night and morning, care could be effective."

Givanni's attack on dental disease is simple. If you have a fungus infection between the toes, common sense tells you to clean the area. But for many people this basic message has never traveled from the feet to the mouth.

The prime killer of teeth is the "no man's land" between them. Trapped food promotes infection and toxins that attack the enamel. Equally important, it destroys the tough periodontal fibers that cement the teeth in place. That's why most people over 30 lose teeth because of diseased gums.

How can you keep your teeth a lifetime? I'd agree with Amos and Andy, it's wise to see the dentist twice a year. But don't expect unrealistic miracles from him. To maintain a healthy mouth you must do most of the work. There are several common-sense ways to accomplish it.

A good dental pack would never separate the teeth from the gums. It should include a soft brush that won't injure tissues and information on how to brush the teeth correctly. Most people just brush the outside surface. You should also clean inside surfaces and your tongue. It also pays dividends to keep an extra toothbrush at work.

Never neglect Givanni's idea. Use dental floss to protect the weakest part of the teeth. Moving this fine thread up and down between the teeth removes newly formed plaque. Plaque consists of food, saliva, and bacteria. It sticks to the teeth every day and generates tooth decay.

In my opinion, the most practical way to remove particles between teeth is by using *stimudents*. These soft triangular wooden toothpicks open up natural pathways between the teeth and give them breathing space. Regular use of stimudents would result in a massive decrease in dental disease. Try the following test if you're not convinced. Give the teeth a good brushing. Then follow with the use of a stimudent. You'll be surprised at the food particles the stimudent removes.

Remember it's easy and expensive to have dentures by 30. Tooth decay tends to run in families. It's usually the result of bathing the teeth continually in sugar cereals, sweet rolls, candy, gum, and sugar snacks between meals or before bedtime, as well as being lazy about mouth hygiene.

Be prepared to pay for preventive dentistry. Adequate cleaning of the teeth by either the dentist or his assistant takes time. If it's neglected or done quickly and superficially, you're in the wrong office.

Perhaps one of the major toothpaste companies will finally promote the total package of preventive dentistry. It would help to stop the "drill and bill" routine in dental offices. And it would be a refreshing change to learn the true facts on TV. Considering today's sophisticated consumer it might even be good for business.

Root Canal Therapy

A horse's shoe can help you make the right decision about your teeth. When your dentist says, "I can extract the tooth or do a root canal operation," how do you reply? When you're sitting in a dental chair with a painfully swollen face, the decision becomes doubly difficult. It's easy to make the wrong choice if you forget about the horse's shoe.

Think about what caused this dilemma in the first place. Usually infection has seeped under an old filling into the pulp of the tooth, which contains blood vessels and nerves. Or perhaps through a crack in the tooth enamel. Or a blow to the tooth has obstructed the blood supply. Eventually infection spreads to the root of the tooth, causing an apical abscess. Like an inflamed appendix, the pulp and nerves then must be removed, or the whole tooth extracted.

Root canal procedures are surrounded by misconceptions. Often people wail, "Don't ever agree to a root canal. They're awfully painful. They rarely work. And you'll end up losing the tooth anyway." Or as one dentist told me, "It's a good approach for the front teeth. But molars have too many roots. It's wiser to extract molars."

The horse's shoe provides an answer. George Herbert in 1640 wrote that, "For want of a nail, the horse's shoe was lost. For want of a shoe, the horse was lost. For want of a horse, the rider was lost. For want of a rider the battle was lost. And for want of a battle the kingdom was lost." Similarly, one dental problem often leads to another, sometimes worse. So never part with a tooth lightly.

Pulling out the abscessed tooth is the old-time remedy. It provides speedy relief. But the extraction of a tooth leaves a gap. Like the lost nail in a horse's shoe, it often triggers a series of other troubles.

A gap in the gum means opposing teeth have nothing to support them during chewing. They, too, become loose and more susceptible to decay. An upper tooth will slowly fall into the hole, or a remaining tooth drift out of position, disturbing the normal bite. The loss of a tooth means more than just the loss of a tooth.

The root canal operation, unlike an appendectomy, requires several steps. The dentist initially removes the nerves in the root. This relieves the pain and drains the abscess. After inflammation has simmered down, the major work is begun. The dentist carefully reams out the roots of the tooth, sterilizes the cavity, then fills the root canals with sealant. Later a sturdy cap is placed over the tooth to provide support.

Don't be an impatient patient if you agree to a root canal procedure. The speedy removal of a gallbladder or appendix provides an immediate recovery. But weeks or months may be needed to determine the outcome of a root canal operation.

Root canal work removes only the infected pulp and nerves. Once this primary site of infection is excised, the residual inflammation around the tooth's root normally settles down. But if the jawbone sustains a long-standing infection, the pain may continue. Then an operation to trim the root of the tooth may be advised to rid the jaw of stubborn inflammation. But there's no point in placing an expensive cap over the tooth until it's confirmed that the root canal treatment has been a success.

Root canal work isn't practical for all patients. If dental care has been neglected for years, the rest of the teeth and gums are probably in terrible shape. It makes little sense to rebuild one tooth in this case. In some patients the root may be fractured or the canal so narrow that even the smallest instruments will not penetrate it.

Time may also be a vital factor. If the patient is awaiting open heart surgery, localized infection must be quickly eradicated. The abscessed tooth must be extracted to speed up the preparation for surgery. It's better to have a live patient without teeth than a dead one with beautifully restored ones.

Who should perform these operations? Whether you're arranging for a new muffler on your car or a root canal procedure on your teeth, the same principle applies. Practice makes perfect.

General dentists who have taken root canal training are available. But endodontists who specialize in this work will achieve better results than dentists who do only an occasional root canal. And remember you can't expect as good a result in a molar tooth with several roots as in a forward tooth with a single root. But in good hands the overall success rate is 90 percent.

Is it worth the inconvenience and expense? Root canal work won't save a kingdom. But it does prevent a hazardous gap in the mouth and a host of other problems. And, like neglecting a horse's shoe, neglect of a tooth will trigger more trouble later on. I'd remind skeptics that few other things in life give 90 percent results or are accomplished with practically no pain.

Wisdom Teeth: To Pull or Not to Pull

Arabic wisdom counsels, "Never trouble trouble until trouble troubles you." But is this sage advice when it comes to wisdom teeth? Failure to extract third molars can be like sitting on a time-bomb. But it's also a major operation, and no one wants the cure to be worse than the disease. As Shakespeare would say, "To pull or not to pull, that is the question."

The person who said, "We ain't what we used to be," could have had the human jaw in mind. Life used to be tough when the jaw worked overtime to chew hard foods. Today's supermarkets, refrigeration, and softer foods have made life easier for the jaw. The result? It's become smaller over the years. This often means insufficient room for wisdom teeth to develop.

Arabic wisdom is preferable on occasion—when the third molar has completely erupted in a normal position and can be cleaned easily. This tooth is valuable, particularly when an opposing molar is also present. They will assist mastication for many years. Normally positioned wisdom teeth can also prove valuable later in life. The second molar may be lost by this time. Then the wisdom tooth may be used for the support of bridgework.

What if the third molar hasn't erupted above the gum? Here there is a difference in opinion. If it is not causing pressure on the second molar, or if there's no evidence of cyst formation, many believe it reasonable to leave it alone. This tooth may still be in place at the age of 90.

But there's also a situation when the buried wisdom tooth becomes a dental time-bomb. For instance, there is a developmental sac around the crown of the unerupted tooth that can become an infected cyst. If this happens, the tooth should be removed.

Buried wisdom teeth can also cause excessive pressure on the adjoining second molars, gradually destroying their roots. Or they can produce undue pressure on the mandibular nerve, resulting in neuralgic pain or tingling sensations of the jaw. There's no point in waiting until this condition destroys the second molar. Another point to remember about wisdom teeth—they should be either totally buried or completely erupted. Partial development is always potential trouble. If the second molar prevents further eruption, infection of either the overlying or the adjacent gum tissue is almost a certainty. Then the chance of losing the second molar from spreading infection is too great. Don't argue when the dentist advises removal of this wisdom tooth.

Over-eruption is also a problem. An excessively high third molar prevents proper occlusion of the other teeth. Such teeth are more likely to develop pyorrhea and are better removed.

Technical reasons may suggest removal of a wisdom tooth. If the lack of space makes it hard to get at the wisdom tooth with a toothbrush, it will surely develop large cavities.

The removal of the tooth can be as easy as rolling off a log, but it can also be a tedious technical operation. I vividly recall having one removed during my premedical years. I thought the dentist's hammering would break my jaw. And, in fact, this can happen. But today new high-speed drills make this less likely.

Removal of the wisdom teeth causes post-operative swelling of the face. Sometimes the edema is so extensive that it alarms the patients, but it is usually not important unless it is associated with a high temperature. There may also be difficulty opening the jaw for a few days.

The cure is rarely worse than the disease. But occasionally when too much bone is destroyed during extraction, the second molar will end up with inadequate support. At other times the root of the tooth is so close to the maxillary sinus that the sinus is affected. Molars of the lower jaw also sit close to the mandibular nerve; difficult extractions can injure this nerve, resulting in either temporary or permanent loss of sensation to the lower jaw.

I agree with Dr. John E. Speck, professor of periodontics at the University of Toronto. He says, "To suggest removing all third molars routinely is roughly comparable to saying everyone's appendix should be removed because they might cause trouble."

Dental Rust: The Big Killer of Teeth

People have the wrong idea about rust. Most of us think it just causes holes in drainpipes, but rust is the main cause of lost teeth in people over the age of 35. It's the reason why more than half of those over 64 years of age are devoid of all teeth. Why has this problem remained an epidemic for centuries? And can North Americans avoid this disease when many dentists are also afflicted with dental rust, better known as periodontal gum disease (PGD)?

Dentistry has made tremendous strides in recent years. Tooth decay can progress to a major extent, yet now the tooth can often be saved. However, there's no way to save a tooth if the cement that holds it in place has been destroyed.

Periodontal disease is an insidious process. In its early stages the gum turns from a natural pink colour to red. Later small spaces form between the gum and the tooth. This condition is called gingivitis—it's not usually painful and can remain unnoticed for many years. But gingivitis usually progresses to periodontitis. The gum starts to pull away from the crown and root of the tooth, causing deep pockets to form where bacteria accumulate and gradually destroy the firm, cement-like structures supporting the tooth.

The main culprit in this disease is a bacterium that deposits rust (plaque) around the base of the teeth. It's a sticky substance that gradually hardens into calculus (tartar). The more calculus, the greater the wedge that pries the tooth from the gum and other support. Dentists treat severe periodontal disease by cutting open the pockets and cleaning out the diseased material. Nature can do remarkable things when the infection is cleared up. In other instances deep scaling by a hygienist every few months can be an alternative to surgery. But the best treatment is preventing periodontal disease from reaching this point.

Some medical consumers might say it's impossible when they consider this fact. In 1972 a number of dentists attending the annual meeting of the American Dental Association were examined by a fellow dentist. He reported that just 5 percent of the dentists' mouths were healthy; 35 percent had gingivitis and 60 percent periodontal disease with pockets of pus.

But don't toss up your hands in despair. Remember that dentists are also human. Some have not learned their own lessons. Others insult their mouths day after day with tobacco or are too lazy to spend some time on good dental hygiene. Common sense, not a dental degree, is the best weapon to fight rusting teeth.

Periodontal gum disease cannot be stopped until people get rid of misconceptions about dental care. It takes more than a visit to the dentist twice a year to prevent PGD and more than just brushing the teeth in the morning and at bedtime.

Some patients form rust around the teeth as others develop dandruff. If that's the case, you must see the hygienist every few months for scaling. And if your dentist cleans your teeth in five minutes, find another one.

It's scrupulous daily dental hygiene, between visits to the dentist, that is the cornerstone of prevention. This means brushing your teeth after every meal or snack, keeping a toothbrush in the office to use after the noon lunch. Laziness and inconsistency are the primary causes of dental rust.

For example, how many people bother to brush the gums on the tongue side of their teeth? Gums, like muscles, need stimulation to keep them firm and adherent to the teeth. So buy a curved toothbrush such as the Reach type to remove the rust on both sides of the teeth.

Some dentists advocate the use of hydrogen peroxide or salt solutions for the gum margins, or moistening the toothbrush with baking soda to improve the health of the gums. Others stress the use of fluoride or antibiotic mouthwashes as a means of cutting down on plaque-forming bacteria. But I question the wisdom of using antibiotics for long periods of time.

Don't forget that it's not only time and money that is at stake when you get lazy with dental hygiene. Teeth are important for both functional and psychological reasons. They play a major role in nutrition, speech, and facial structure. They affect how you look and how you relate to others. Most people fail to realize the importance of teeth until they're extracted.

4

Sports and Exercise

The Boston Marathon and "Ego Infarction"

I recently heard an intriguing story during a trip to Boston, where I was revisiting medical centers where I trained for several years. At such medical reunions many tales are swapped over lunch. One story in particular drove home a message about heart disease and how people react to the threat of impending death.

Doctors had informed a patient that his three coronary arteries were practically blocked. They strongly advised coronary bypass surgery. But the patient refused. Instead, he lost 37 pounds, started a vigorous exercise program, and eventually ran in the Honolulu Marathon. Later still, in 90° heat, he tackled the Boston Marathon. Newspapers proclaimed loudly how he had defied doctors and medical science.

One thing wasn't printed in the papers. During the Honolulu race the man suffered chest pain for six hours. But the next day he began training for another marathon. Many days later an electrocardiogram showed he had suffered a coronary attack during the Honolulu Marathon. Yet this man is still training for races.

You have to give him top marks for trying, and he may even be winning the battle. But he is one of many patients who overdo things following a coronary. Some are not so fortunate and die from strenuous activity.

The crushing pain of heart attack causes different psychological reactions. It's impossible to have the threat of impending doom hanging over you without reacting to it in some way. In effect a myocardial infarction is always accompanied by "ego infarction."

Patients worry about job security, loss of earning power, and how their sex life, drinking, smoking, and other pleasures will be affected. Can life ever be the same again? Few patients leave hospital without some degree of homecoming depression.

Patients cope with this threat to life and self-esteem in various ways. Denial is the most common reaction. One study revealed that 20 percent of patients refused to believe the diagnosis three weeks after a proven heart attack. Others, such as the marathon runner, simply overdo it. Some take the opposite tack and quit living. It's a good excuse to retire honorably from all the traumas of life. I asked heart specialists and psychiatrists how to temper the effects of ego infarction. What they advised sounds sensible for most of us.

First of all, everyone has to accept a certain amount of anxiety as a normal component of a heart attack. There's always a degree of self-pity and apprehension about the future. Drugs can help to soften this reaction.

But one point that is particularly important. Understanding this fact could save some needless worry. A follow-up of coronary patients revealed that weakness was the most distressing symptom. Some patients felt great while in hospital but on returning home just walking the length of the house caused severe exhaustion. You may ask, "What's so earth-shaking about that? Surely it's normal to be weak after a heart attack." You're right, but there's more than meets the eye here.

If you ever suffer a heart attack, remember this. Bed rest causes a loss of 10 to 15 percent of your strength per week because of muscle atrophy. It also results in a 25 percent decrease in the oxygen uptake by the body.

Investigators in Dallas, Texas, dramatically illustrated this fact. Two trained athletes volunteered to spend three weeks in bed. Then they underwent a series of tests. It required a month for them to regain their original strength. It's the bed, not the heart, that produces much of the weakness.

What's the best antidote for physical and psychological problems following a coronary? The Boston doctors strongly advised getting patients out of bed at the earliest possible time. Then not waiting too long to return them to bed for normal sexual activities.

Regrettably, some patients become cardiac cripples. One doctor admitted that he had become a basket case. He would lie in bed with his stethoscope and listen to his heart for hours on end.

I wouldn't advise anyone with known heart disease to tackle the Boston Marathon. Nor would I suggest he take the advice of Robert Hutchins who said, "Whenever I feel like exercise I lie down until the feeling passes." I think moderate exercise is the answer. As John Racine said in 1668, "He who wishes to travel far spares his mount."

Buy Running Shoes to Fight Depression

How can everyone ignore such an obvious medical way to relieve mental stress? Year after year tons of drugs are given to depressed patients. Yet Dr. Hans Selye's experiments indicate there's a simple, cheap, effective way to fight mental illness. Dr. Selye was President of the International Institute of Stress at the University of Montreal and one of the world's renowned scientists. His basic experiments should be heeded by psychiatrists, governments, and the rest of us. It could save people and this country millions of dollars.

Dr. Selye subjected 10 sedentary rats to electric shock treatments, blinding lights, and deafening noise. In a month they were all dead. Then 10 other rats were toughened up on a treadmill and subjected to the same stress. A month later they were still in good shape.

Athletes always point to the numerous benefits of exercise. The heart muscle strengthens and can pump more blood. The lungs become less emphysematous with aging. The bones remain strong. But what about the brain? Is there a crucial link there that's being neglected?

Dr. Howard L. Hartley, director of the exercise laboratory at the Massachusetts General Hospital, says that strenuous exercise causes changes in the chemistry of the brain in experimental animals. Possibly these alterations also occur in humans. Some researchers believe it's the newly discovered endomorphines that trigger a sense of well-being following exercise.

Professor Robert S. Brown and Dr. John M. Taub of the University of Virginia studied depression in students. During a 10-week period they prescribed jogging five days a week. The researchers found that feelings of anger, hostility, fatigue, and tension all decreased.

Doctors J.H. Greist and J.T. Faris of the University of Wisconsin carried out a similar study with the same result. It confirmed that depressed people feel better when they run. The dark clouds lift and tensions simmer down.

Therapists started these experimental sessions with stretching exercises and then 30 to 45 minutes of walking and running. During jogging the patients talked about the weather, running gear, or different routes. But discussion never touched on depression. The therapists noted that patients never seemed depressed when exercising. The last group consisted of 30 people, and 24 quickly recovered from depression. Four of the six who failed to improve never became runners.

Running out of a depression has a bonus. It's a do-it-yourself form of therapy. Patients discover there's no overpowering need to load their systems with drugs. They happily experience new bodily sensations while jogging and learn their illness is self-limiting and can be defeated.

Exercise, like any other treatment, isn't a panacea for all types of depression. But for most cases of mild to moderate depression there's ample evidence that it's superior to drugs in elevating the mood and relaxing the patient. And it has none of the side effects.

Sir William Osler made a sage remark many years ago. He reminded doctors that, when several treatments are available for an illness, that suggests none are very effective. Today there are dozens of antidepressant pills on the market. But psychotherapy and drugs only help about 25 percent of patients. So why not try running shoes?

On checking Canadian hospitals, however, I found none that used this therapy. I asked why not. Several psychiatrists replied they had never thought about it. Some were concerned that patients might get into trouble running around city streets. And one annoyed doctor said he didn't study medicine to supervise a physical training program! Yet several thought they would give it a try.

Most psychiatric nurses felt it would be good for their patients. The general consensus was that too many patients sit around psychiatric units doing nothing, or merely stare at TV all day. Life becomes too soft and easy for them.

And a few of these patients use their depression to get out of working. As one nurse remarked, "If we requested that these people clean the washrooms every day, many would quickly get over their depression."

Perhaps what's been proven good for rats also makes sense for humans. After all, if jogging is good for the healthy mind, surely it would also help to lubricate a troubled one.

Winston Churchill once said, "Too many people were a hulk, only breathing and excreting." In 1980 too many North Americans inside and outside of psychiatric units are in that category. Exchanging pills for running shoes might be a good way to fight depression and also improve lifestyle.

Unsuspected Hazards For Joggers

"Don't you think you're overdoing it? Pushing your luck too far? Moderation is always wiser." I was giving advice to one of my sons who had developed a questionable habit. He doesn't drink too much or drive too fast. But for exercise he runs up the 37 floors of his apartment building. Not once but twice. And I had just read an intriguing article explaining why some healthy young joggers suddenly collapse and die. It should be required reading for everyone who exercises strenuously.

The article by Dr. Azorides R. Morales appeared in the May 1981 issue of *Executive Health*. He's a professor of pathology at the University of Miami and he describes himself as a cautious jogger. For good reason. He and his colleagues have discovered that exercise can sometimes lead to death for unsuspected reasons. He suggests this can be avoided.

The pathologists performed autopsies on two people who died while exercising. One was a 34-year-old male jogger. Another was a 17-year-old girl who died while swimming. The pathologists expected to find atherosclerosis, particularly in the 34-year-old man. But they found little or none.

What they did find in these cases was a bridged left coronary artery. Two coronary arteries, the left and right, feed oxygenated blood to the heart muscle. The left coronary artery carries 85 percent of the blood that nourishes the heart. It also supplies the largest part of the heart, the left ventricle. This chamber sends out blood to the entire body.

The major branches of the coronary arteries normally run over the surface of the heart. Smaller branches then descend into the heart muscle to supply it with energy.

But some joggers have a potential problem. The major branches are surrounded on part of their route by the heart muscle. Pathologists refer to this abnormality as "bridging."

Dr. Azorides Morales says bridging isn't a new discovery. Since the 1920s studies in several countries have shown a degree of coronary artery bridging present in about one quarter of all hearts. But no one has previously suggested this is a cause of sudden death.

So why don't more joggers die from coronary artery bridging? The degree of bridging is the answer, and whether the surrounding arteries are reduced in size and number as a result. This combination occurs in about one person in 200.

How bridging kills joggers and swimmers can be logically explained. Diastole is the heart's resting phase. Eighty percent of blood reaching the heart muscle flows through the coronary arteries while the heart relaxes.

During systole, the heart muscle and muscle bridges contract. This squeezing reduces the amount of blood flowing through the coronary arteries. At the normal heart rate of 72 beats a minute, a reduced supply of oxygenated blood doesn't affect heart function.

But if you're out of shape and the rate increases to 150 a minute, this can tip the scale. Since the heart is working harder, the relaxation phase is shortened. Now only 50 percent of the blood goes through the coronaries during diastole. At a time when the muscle urgently needs more oxygen, muscular bridges are decreasing the blood supply.

The presence of bridging becomes more important in older joggers. Atherosclerosis is more likely to be present as well. These fatty deposits partially block the coronary vessels. Bridging and atherosclerosis then become a lethal combination. Autopsies reveal that even prior to death, victims of this disorder usually suffer several minute heart attacks.

How do joggers know if they have bridging? At the moment it can be demonstrated only by special x-ray techniques. But this procedure also carries a risk. Currently there's no practical way to detect this anatomical defect.

Jogging, like medication, requires careful titration. Too much or too little is dangerous. Be sure to build up fitness gradually. And don't forget the danger number is 150. It appears that damage to the heart occurs when the pulse rate reaches or exceeds 150 beats per minute.

Hearts in good condition don't have to beat at a rapid rate. A marathoner's pulse rarely exceeds 120. But what about the rate during the run up 37 floors? Such data isn't available in medical journals. My son, however, provided the answer. "130," he said, "and stop worrying."

Which is the more educational? The after-dinner lecture, or the pre-dinner cocktail hour? I find that it's often the conviviality of the cocktail hour that brings the real story out. Recently a visiting professor gave an after-dinner lecture on the latest methods of diagnosing and treating jogging injuries. But what he told me in conversation before the meal was more enlightening. He revealed that he had failed to follow his own advice. His error had crippled him, and the rest of us can learn from his misfortune.

The professor appeared to be in prime condition. Why shouldn't he be? Until recently he had run 60 miles every week. But now he admitted to severe pain in his leg joints, severe enough that he had to get out of a car every 40 miles or so. Worse still, he could no longer play his favorite sport, squash, due to damaged knees.

Like millions of other North Americans the professor started running for its physical and psychological benefits. But he had joined the 60 percent of runners who eventually sustain injuries that prevent them from running. The cause is no great mystery. Runners simply overuse the joints.

Few joggers realize the immense force that is at work in this exercise. The impact of jogging results in 10 times the body's weight being applied to the joints. It's estimated that a typical distance runner doing 130 kilometers a week subjects the joints to 40,000 impacts. Hundreds of miles and millions of heel and joint strikes later, joggers are often brought to their knees.

For years health authorities have preached the virtues of jogging. Now I hear a subdued warning from these same people. One orthopedic surgeon told me, "The potential for injury is so great that for preventive medical reasons I advise patients not to jog."

A U.S. surgeon remarked, "Don't get me wrong. Regular exercise is a must for good health. But I can no longer accept a 60 percent risk of injury for jogging. Other sports such as swimming, bicycling, and walking do not involve this huge risk."

Dr. Charles Godfrey, head of rehabilitation at Toronto's Wellesley Hospital, revealed a significant appraisal of running. He stated, "There is a constant bemusement on my part by the fervor of the gasping masses. It's a sort of 'I believe in the Father, the Son, and the Holy Ghost—and Adidas!'"

This blind faith that all will be well results in an endless list of orthopedic injuries. Some runners suffer from hamstring muscle pain, lumbosacral strain, and achilles tendonitis. Older joggers sustain stress fractures of the feet and pelvic bones as their skeletal structures become thinner. Women are prone to jogger's nipple from the friction of clothes. And there is at least one case of penile frostbite.

Can running circumvent your becoming a medical statistic? One authority suggested a logical first step. "You don't paint over dirt and rust," he said, "so if you're 50 pounds overweight, lose this before you hit the pavement." Most injuries occur when new converts try to do too much too soon. All the experts agree that would-be joggers should do a pile of walking as a prelude to running. If you're 40 or older, walk an hour every day for several months.

Don't make the professor's mistake. He repeatedly damaged his knees trying to continue long-distance running. Over and over again he endured pain in the joints. But he refused to give up running long enough to allow his knees to recover. You cannot run your way out of an injury. This approach merely exchanges a minor problem for a major one.

Running, like high diving or skiing, is not for everyone. After all, how many of us have the ideal weight of 135 pounds and height of five feet seven inches for this sport? But if you can't rid yourself of the compulsion, at least purchase well-constructed shoes that help cushion the blows.

Tread carefully if you have a shaky marriage. Sociologists report that some jogging wives begin to reject a husband whose main occupation is watching TV.

Or jogging husbands look for another partner who will measure up to their macho image.

Angry runners will remind me of other sporting injuries. Recently three male athletes between the ages of 25 and 50 noticed an increased desire to urinate. But they had trouble emptying the bladder. The reason? They had all been cycling for long distances on hard, narrow seats. Prolonged pressure on the prostate gland had triggered the problem. Another cyclist developed a twisted testicle on a long trip. Alas, there seems to be no foolproof sport.

But I think the professor's injury gives pause for thought. I may end up breaking my leg on the tennis court. But there's a good chance it will heal and give me another day on the court. The professor will never jog again. Anyone for tennis?

Who Says Tennis Can't Compete with Jogging?

Do you get tired of people preaching to you about the virtues of jogging? That it's the be-all and end-all for a healthy heart? That tennis may be fun, but doesn't improve cardiovascular health? Well, I've been waiting a long time for researchers to set die-hard joggers back on their heels. And I hope they take my advice and buy a mirror.

Dr. Barry W. Ramo, a cardiologist in Albuquereque, and Daniel F. Friedman at Duke University recently reported in *Physician and Sportsmedicine* on the cardiovascular health of the average tennis player.

These researchers studied 28 men ranging in age from 45 to 72 years. All 28 played tennis year round and were either intermediate or intermediate advanced club players. None was a tournament champion, nor did any have a history of heart or lung disease.

The subjects were divided into two groups. Group A were between 45 and 55 years of age. Group B were between 56 and 72 years of age. Like many other tennis players their health habits were very inconsistent. Five members of group A and six of group B had smoked 20 cigarettes a day for at least 20 years. Five were still smoking at the time of the study. And four of the players were 20 percent overweight.

The younger players were on the tennis court an average of six hours a week, which constituted 80 percent of their total exercise. The older ones played an average of 10 hours every week, which amounted to 97 percent of their total exercise.

Dr. Ramo and Friedman conducted the study during the summer to determine the effects of temperature on the heart. Players were examined at midday or late in the afternoon. The average temperature was 35.1° C, with temperatures ranging from 23.9° C to 40.0° C. Electrocardiograms (ECGs) were taken of the heart before, during, and 30 to 60 minutes after a singles game of tennis.

What did the study show? All 28 players achieved heart rates greater than

60 percent of their predicted maximum capacity. But 24 of the 28 had mean heart rates between 70 and 90 percent of the predicted maximum capacity. The heart rates returned to normal in an average of 20 minutes.

The electrocardiograms showed that the heart's rhythm is affected by tennis. Two of the young and four of the older players had premature ventricular contractions before the start of the game. But five of the young and all but three of the older players developed these extra heartbeats during the game. At no time did the electrocardiogram detect any deficiency of blood going to the heart's muscle.

How does the heat affect the heart? My family often remind me that, "Only mad dogs and Englishmen go out in the noonday sun." This study revealed that the heart showed no significant changes between extremes of temperature.

But does tennis help to condition the heart? The results showed that the heart rates were high enough to have a beneficial effect. And here's one point I don't want joggers to miss. In spite of the start and stop nature of tennis, the heart rate nevertheless achieved a steady level. Jogging, cycling, and swimming are not the only routes to cardiovascular health.

There's more good news for tennis players. Drs. P.A. Volk and W.M. Savin conducted tests to determine the amount of oxygen consumed during various sports. Their conclusion? Middle-aged men whose only form of exercise is tennis use the same amount of oxygen as males of the same age who have jogged 24 kilometers a week for the last 10 years.

What's my advice to joggers? The next time you start off on a long run, take a mirror with you. Then take a look at your tortured expression every few miles. I think the intelligent *Homo sapiens* might then ask himself, "Why should I ruin my knees and endure such pain when I can buy a tennis racket and have some fun?" But I know I won't convince determined joggers. For such diehards, however, I have a list of good orthopedic surgeons!

Skiers Should Heed Ellison's Law

Art Ellison, an orthopedic surgeon and former classmate of mine, has credentials that read like a *Who's Who* in international skiing. He is the physician for the U.S. National Ski team and chief of sports medicine at the University of Massachusetts Medical School. And he's noted for Ellison's Law: "He who does not fall down rarely gets hurt."

Recreational skiers should develop a healthy respect for this rule. Even for those who are not mathematically inclined, the accident figures are impressive. This winter 12,000,000 North Americans will ascend slopes with skis. Over 300,000 of them will descend in ski patrol toboggans.

The psychiatrist's office may be the place to prevent some injuries. The desire to speed down a snow-covered hill at 60 mph on two thin pieces of wood without preliminary training needs examination.

Yet one study revealed that 75 percent of those injured had not received ski instruction. That's why Ellison told me, "Now I spend most of my time rebuilding the wounded knees of skiers." He says about 30 percent of all ski accidents are either knee ligament injuries or fractures of the tibia.

Novice skiers are a hazard on the slopes. It's startling to read that first-day beginners account for 6 percent of all broken bones. They are also three times more likely to get hurt than experts. Ski jumping has a surprisingly low rate of injury. This is because the jumper is superbly trained.

Today there's a similarity between skiing and airports. With millions of skiers on the hills, there's an increasing number of collisions and near misses. A study in Vermont revealed that 12.5 percent of the accidents resulted from collisions. Some people hit other skiers. Others smashed into trees, slalom gates, and lift towers. Defensive skiing, like defensive driving, is one way to stay alive.

How can you remain on skis rather than on crutches? Remember that skiing is an intense, demanding sport that requires strength and sudden muscle contraction. Unfortunately, most skiers try to ski themselves into shape. Recreational skiers are therefore more likely to be injured in the late afternoon of the first two days of skiing. Many admit they were simply too tired to avert a fall that led to trouble. Loss of control is the major cause of skiing accidents.

Improve your muscle power for skiing before the season begins. Jogging and indoor rope jumping increase strength, agility, and timing. You can also toughen the thigh muscles by extending the leg with increasing weights over the ankles or by jumping over progressively larger objects.

What about food? Can the right diet decrease the possibility of injury? We know that the body consumes large amounts of carbohydrates during downhill skiing. Moreover, researchers taking biopsies of muscles have shown that the carbohydrate content of the muscles declines during a week of skiing. They believe this glycogen depletion may explain why so many injuries happen at the end of the day.

The Swedish ski team examined these findings and changed their eating habits. Coaches now give them a high carbohydrate meal the evening before competition. It takes between 8 to 12 hours to replenish glycogen stores.

Recreational skiers should also maintain high levels of carbohydrate. Don't concentrate just on steaks at the ski lodge. Make sure you also consume bread, spaghetti, pancakes, and other rich carbohydrate foods.

Regrettably, skiers can't eat their way out of one cause of injury. Forty percent of leg injuries result from failure of bindings to release from skis. No one has yet invented the perfect binding, but there are some sound ways to decrease the chance of this accident.

First, be sure bindings are good ones, fit properly, and are in good working order. A dramatic rise in ski injuries to children suggests that borrowed or rented equipment that is ill-fitting is to blame. The binding, like any machine with moving parts, must be frequently cleaned and lubricated. Be sure to remove dirt that might affect performance. Watch out for loose mounting. And cover up bindings when transporting them on the outside of a car. This will protect them from road salt spray.

Tests on seven popular bindings showed one universal problem. They were all sensitive to freezing. This can even occur while the skier rides a chair lift. Skiers should routinely open and close bindings to remove ice and learn how to perform the self-release test to check the correct setting of the binding. Experts say that most beginners wear the binding too tight.

Another expert advises, "Skiers should know their own limitations, their equipment, and the sport." Recognize signs of fatigue. These precautions will ensure safe, happy skiing. And don't forget Ellison's Law.

Sport Injuries: An Ounce of Prevention

Can a simple charley horse cause permanent, disabling injury to a young athlete? Can you prevent an injured knee from developing chronic trouble? Can players avert catastrophic injuries? I asked these questions recently at the new Bobby Orr Sports Therapy Centre at York University in Toronto.

It's an impressive complex with indoor and outdoor running tracks, swimming pool, basketball courts, gymnasium, and other facilities. But the prime reason for its existence is the treatment and prevention of sports injuries. I learned there are still many misconceptions about sporting accidents and that some injuries are like an elephant's memory.

Ed Nowalkoski, head therapist, hammered home an important message: "Don't let small injuries become big ones. It happens over and over again. And it's a tragedy when it strikes a young and promising athlete."

How can it happen today with so much medical knowledge and fitness awareness? An example is the common charley horse resulting from a blow to the thigh. Frequently people discount it, saying, "Oh, he's just got a charley horse."

But that morning in the clinic I saw a young boy who had suffered this injury. No one was treating it lightly anymore. I could feel the underlying thigh muscle grinding as the leg moved. It was a classic case of mismanagement.

This teenager had sustained a major blow to the thigh during a hockey game. His coach sent him home with instructions to apply cold and then heat. No one had examined him the days that followed. He hobbled around, believing he was getting better.

During this time blood collected deep in the quadriceps muscle. At this crucial point the blood should have been aspirated with a needle, a simple task. Instead, the blood became calcified scar tissue, eventually destroying muscle tissue and normal function. This vital muscle can never be restored. And any degree of loss will impede the professional dreams of an athlete.

Another important point was made, one that eluded me in medical school.

The knee is like an elephant, I was told. It never forgets an injury. Why? Because ligaments of the knee joint become lax after trauma. This produces increased mobility of the joint, which in turn leads to further problems.

Fifty percent of sport injuries involve the knee. Trouble usually begins with a slight twisting of the joint. The athlete may miss a couple of games, then return with a looser knee joint. Often it's injured again and the vicious cycle begins.

Athletes should be helped to avoid this pitfall and encouraged to undertake remedial exercises to build up muscles around the knee. These will compensate for the weakened ligaments and decrease the chance of repetitive injury. Stable knees are vital to participation in sports. We've lost the thrill of Bobby Orr on ice because of unstable knees.

The Bobby Orr Centre stresses a team approach in treating injuries. Coaches, sports therapists, family doctors, and orthopedic surgeons all assess an accident quickly and start an immediate program of treatment. Often delays are the cause of chronic disability.

But prevention is always better than cure. And good conditioning is the way to avoid injury. After all, it's strength that averts accidents, so don't try to play yourself into shape. You may be injured before you reach that goal. And it could be a catastrophic accident.

For instance, during the last 45 years 646 athletes have died from head and neck injuries. In addition hundreds of athletes are paralyzed every football season. Players can forestall some of these disastrous injuries by doing preseason neck exercises. Strengthening the neck muscles will provide added insurance for the spinal cord. We all know it's surrounded by bony vertebrae. But few athletes realize the vulnerability of this structure. For example, a 25-cent piece dropped from a height of 15 inches onto exposed spinal cord will completely and permanently destroy all nerve function.

The Bobby Orr Therapy Centre agrees that common sense prevents injury. Therapists there would tell you not to use the head and neck as a battering ram in football just because you're wearing a helmet. And why lose an eye playing hockey when wire mesh face protectors are available? Or suffer the same accident skiing when shatter-proof goggles can be purchased for a few dollars?

They also warn athletes of new sports injuries. For instance, ophthalmologists are seeing more eyes damaged in tennis and squash. With squash balls traveling at 100 mph, a simple eye protector can save a lifetime's vision.

The American Occupational Safety and Health Administration issued a startling statement a few years ago. They calculated that football players, whether high school, college, or professional, had a 200 times greater chance of injury than coal miners. Dr. Harley G. Feldick, team physician and director of student health at the University of Iowa, says, "If we don't change the game, we may not have a game to play."

What makes coal mining safer than contact sports? Harvard psychiatrist

Chester M. Pierce says, "In football the contract is either you hurt the opponent or he hurts you. The coach must have his men feeling that they not only can kill, but that they should kill."

Thomas Tutko, a psychologist at San Jose State University in California, made another interesting comment. He remarked that, "Too often athletics have become a direct substitute for war."

But do parents want coaches to make war with their children? Or to teach them skills that mean spending the rest of their days as quadriplegics in wheelchairs?

Here's a prime example of what coaches shouldn't teach. The hard plastic football helmet was developed as a major breakthrough in safety. But paradoxically this design has increased the number of head and neck injuries. Some coaches think more about winning than wheelchairs. Formerly they taught players to use the shoulders and body block. But with the advent of the hard helmet, they seized the opportunity to use the head as a battering ram. No one knows how many quadriplegics are now paralyzed due to this change in tactics. And in spite of warnings by doctors, some coaches still persist in this practice. I talked to several coaches and players who said, "The head block has just become a part of the game."

So has violence. The May 1977 issue of *Physicians and Sportsmedicine* had some chilling facts on how fans generate much of the trouble. In Italy a rugby player had part of his ear bitten off. In Guatemala angry hometown fans used machetes to kill five members of a winning soccer team. And in the 101st running of the Kentucky Derby hooligans tossed beer cans in the path of the horses as they raced down the backstretch.

Some people laugh it off by saying boys will be boys. They forget it's possible for young people to cause man-sized injuries. Every year about 30 Americans die playing amateur football. And in 1979, 40,000 of the 385,904 interscholastic injuries involved the head and neck.

The situation is the same in Canada. A Royal Commission on violence reached several basic conclusions. Its report stated that violence in hockey now starts at a much younger age. One reason is that TV shows young kids how the professional game is played, violence and all. Yet trying to simulate idols can have disastrous consequences. In Canada, prior to the use of hockey face masks, 40 boys lost an eye every year. And in the U.S., there were 25,000 facial injuries in 1979.

Can parents help to keep children out of wheelchairs? A first step might be the improvement of their own language. Standing on the sidelines yelling "Kill him!" simply adds parental fuel to the fire. Young athletes desperately seek the approval of parents, teachers, and coaches. If violence is encouraged, even vocally, children will try to instigate it. And tragedy will inevitably and needlessly follow.

Parents and safety organizations should also take a hard stand against soft penalties. Violence in contact sports often pays off for a team, producing winning games. Tough penalties could stop it.

But Peter Finch, in the movie *Network*, had the best idea. He shouted to Americans to turn off their TV sets. Television didn't tell them the truth about anything. And it was making them mindless creatures.

I'd like to see the faces of TV sponsors, team owners, coaches, and players when Neilsen ratings for just one major professional game sank to zero. And TV cameras focused on an empty football stadium or a vacant hockey arena.

This one act could change things overnight. It would tell everyone we don't pay good money to watch goon tactics. That we want skilled and classy players to perform without fear of needless injury. And that we want professional athletes to teach our children how to play a fair game. Until that time comes, it will continue to be safer in coal mines.

Motorcyclists: Human Cannonballs?

Are you facing the dilemma of the motorcycle? Does your son feel he can't live without one? Is your daughter riding on the back of one? Should you approve or not? Is it an emotional reaction to decide it's too hazardous a way to travel? Or are motorcyclists unjustifiably branded as the hellions of the road? To reach conclusions for these questions parents and young people should be armed with facts. They could save someone from becoming a human cannonball.

First of all, who is the typical motorcycle accident victim? Statistics claim he's a man in his early 20s. The typical accident occurs on a Saturday or Sunday late in the afternoon. Usually on a dry road without an intersection. The scene is becoming more common every year. In 1978, 166,000 Americans were admitted to hospital for emergency treatment after a motorcycle accident. 4,700 of them died. Many others were crippled for life.

A surgeon who specializes in emergency care told me, "Some of these kids look like ground hamburger when they're brought to us. They've been dragged along the ground for 40 feet with a 500-pound bike on top of them. Or hurled through the air at 60 miles an hour before striking a tree. Anyone who rides a motorbike is a potential human cannonball."

We can expect more of these tragedies. Motorcycle registrations increased from 2.3 to 4.8 million in the U.S. between 1969 and 1978. California now has over 700,000 licensed motorcyclists on the road.

How often this misfortune affects you depends on where you live. In Washington, D.C., it must be hard for parents to sleep at night. Incredibly, there are 916 accidents annually for every 10,000 registrations. Montana is the safest state, with 99 per 10,000. But beautiful Hawaii is the most lethal state; it has 24 deaths per 10,000 motorcycles. North Dakota is the lowest with 3.7 per 10,000.

Is there anything unique about motorcycle injuries? Dr. P. Zettas, an orthopedic surgeon at the Valley Medical Center in Fresno, California, issued a report on these accidents in the November 1979 *Journal of Trauma*. He says that motorcycle injuries are usually complicated by infection. The reason is obvious. Gravel, cinders, grass, glass, or oil enter the wound when a rider is dragged along the ground.

There's another distinguishing effect. Dr. Zettas analyzed 260 consecutive cases of motorcycle injury. Fifty-four percent of the riders suffered broken bones. And many were severe, crushing ones that disrupted the blood supply to bones and joints. This resulted in bones that failed to unite. Six of the riders required lower limb amputations.

Dr. Bahij S. Salibi, chief neurosurgeon at the Marshfield Clinic in Wisconsin, shook his head when I asked about motorcycle accidents. He said, "The worst head injuries I see are those of motorcycle victims. Some are dead on arrival. Others have severe concussions. Still others are left with epileptic seizures or permanent paralysis. And often there's added damage to heart, lungs, liver, spleen, bowel, or bladder."

Not all surgeons damn motorcycles. Dr. R. Cottinham at St. Thomas's Hospital, London, England, lays much of the blame on motorists, especially those who can't see anything on the road that's less than five feet wide. He believes the answer lies in re-educating car drivers and making them more aware of smaller vehicles on the road.

If the motorcycle is a must, how can you decrease the possibility of the driver or rider becoming a human cannonball? The first step is a course in motorcycle safety. The second is sobriety; 40 percent of fatal accidents are due to excessive alcohol consumption.

Never forget that the principle hazard is the automobile. It causes 70 percent of accidents. Some drivers weave down the road drunk. Others suddenly open a car door without looking and knock over a passing motorcyclist. Or emerge from a side road without stopping. Or carelessly cut into the path of an oncoming rider.

Don't neglect the crash helmet. Failure to do so doubles the chance of head injury. And beware of skimpy clothing. Leather jackets, pants, and boots offer protection against lacerations and foot injuries. And bright clothing provides greater visibility to the motorist.

Drive defensively above all else. One must assume that all car drivers are either incompetent, careless, or drunk. This assumption alone will save many young people from becoming human cannonballs.

One final point before you sign the bill of sale. Don't forget it's an imperfect world. There will always be drunken or careless motorists. There'll always be unseen potholes in the road or patches of oil on an already slippery curve. Thin air provides no protection. So motorcycles will remain a dangerous way to travel.

Eye Injuries in Racket Sports

Tennis, squash, and racketball are supposed to be the safe sports, the game for ladies and gentlemen. But some racket-swinging patients these days look like survivors of the Vietnam war. Today millions of North Americans are playing racket games. Thousands, including spectators, lose an eye in the process. It's because the public, and many doctors, are unaware of the hazards of these sports.

Dr. Morton H. Sulenfreund and Dennis B. Freilich of New York sounded an alarm in the 1976 *Journal of the American Medical Association*. They reported that most tennis injuries occur when players rush the net. A 38-year-old physician playing at the net was struck by a tennis ball traveling at 50 miles an hour. The retina of his eye was torn and hemorrhage followed immediately.

The report also mentioned a 33-year-old woman who was merely watching a tennis match. A wild ball struck her in the left eye. Her vision was interrupted immediately by flashes of light and floating particles. Both patients needed surgery to repair detached retinas.

Such reports in medical journals don't receive much attention. But two years later Drs. Paul F. Vinger and Daniel W. Tolpin, both Harvard ophthalmologists, expressed alarm at the explosive growth in the number of eye injuries from racket sports. They estimated that in 1976 there were 3,220 U.S. players who received eye injuries. That in Malaysia badminton was the leading cause of eye injury. And that in Quebec 10 percent of all eye trauma is due to racket sports.

Two Canadian eye specialists, Drs. Michael Easterbrook and Tom Pashby of the University of Toronto, have repeatedly warned of these dangers. In the January 1981 issue of *Physician and Sportsmedicine*, Dr. Easterbrook's message is loud and clear. It's not just the amateurs who get into trouble. Experienced, competitive players are in a higher risk category. They are less willing to give up control of center court. This exposes them to a greater chance of injury from a racket or ball.

One male squash player with 15 years of experience was struck by a racket when his opponent lost his grip. He suffered a fracture of the orbital bone, causing massive hemorrhage into the eye. Another female squash player was also hit by a racket. The blow ruptured supporting structures of the eye lens. Dense hemorrhage resulted in persistent glaucoma and the development of a cataract. The patient lost a major part of her vision.

The same story is repeated in other countries. In one British study, 11 percent of squash injuries to the eye resulted in blindness.

Can such tragedies be prevented? Players must first toss away old misconceptions. For example, players often believe that plastic lenses won't break. Others mistakenly think that prescription lenses with hardened glass are safe. These beliefs leave players exposed with a false sense of security. A 21-year-old male player with hardened lenses was struck by a squash racket. The lens of his glasses shattered on impact into hundreds of pieces. Severe bleeding and a torn retina resulted.

There's only one good preventive method to save eyes in racket sports: The eye guard. But don't scrimp when purchasing one. The rims of some cheaper guards have been known to be driven into players' eyes.

And don't be persuaded to purchase an open eye guard. This type provides no protection from the direct hit of a small ball. In one study, 5 of 67 squash players and nearly half the racketball players suffering eye injuries were wearing open guards.

The closed eye guard provides the best protection. Prescription and non-prescription lenses should be either a CR 39 plastic or polycarbonate plastic with a 3 mm thickness at the center of the lens. The frame should also be strong enough to withstand the force of a ball traveling at 140 miles an hour.

There are some common-sense precautions as well. Dennis Hull, former hockey star of the Chicago Black Hawks, possessed one of the hardest shots in the NHL. I've also seen him drive a tennis ball with incredible force. I never look away for an instant when he's serving. Use the same caution with squash. Injuries happen when squash players turn to see where their opponent is going to hit the ball.

Be especially alert at the start of games. Tennis injuries often occur during warm-up when more than one ball is in play on the same court. And don't slam a ball in anger or frustration after losing a point. Wild balls have caused some severe and unnecessary damage.

A good friend of mine smiles silently when I urge him to wear an eye guard. He's a good young squash player, but wears prescription glasses for short-sightedness. That makes him especially vulnerable. Myopic lenses are thinnest in the center. I've got one last card to play with him. I'm showing him medical pictures of the eye injuries to squash players. They, too, believed they were quicker than the squash ball.

Don't Dive into a Wheelchair This Summer

What a difference a few seconds can make in a life. One moment he was standing on the diving board, healthy, muscular, self-sufficient. Five seconds later he was paralyzed, unable to control urinary or bowel functions, and totally dependent on others for a lifetime. There is no injury more devastating, physically or emotionally, to an individual and his family. Every summer it strikes too many homes.

The reason is that few talk about this problem. Most people discount the possibility of its happening. We often hear of boaters who drown for failing to wear a life-jacket. Others who suffer waterskiing injuries. But we rarely consider the danger lurking below the dark surface of swimming pools or lakes.

Dr. Charles H. Tator, head of the Department of Neurosurgery at Toronto's Western Hospital, studied the spinal cord injuries of patients admitted to two Toronto hospitals over a 25-year period. Traffic accidents and work-related injuries each accounted for about a third of the cases he examined. Fifteen percent were related to sports and recreation accidents; 11 percent of these were due to diving.

Dr. Harry Botterell, one of Canada's most noted neurosurgeons, revealed more shocking news. He told the Annual Meeting of the Royal College of Surgeons in 1975 that 65 percent of acute cord injuries were the result of diving into shallow water. The average patient was 22, and 94 percent were males. The accidents usually occurred in late afternoon or evening.

The extent of paralysis in such cases depends on the severity of location of the injury. The spinal cord is like a telephone cable. If a ditch-digging machine cuts the buried wires, the telephone goes dead. Similarly, if an injury severs the spinal cord at the waist, messages from the brain are interrupted and the legs cannot move (paraplegia). Injury to the cord in the neck results in paralysis of arms, legs, urinary and bowel function (quadriplegia). Even compression of the spinal cord that stops the blood supply for only a few seconds will permanently damage spinal nerves.

Yet the human spine is not injured easily. In 1978 an Air Canada plane crashed during takeoff. The passengers were subjected to a force of 25 Gs on impact, a force three times greater than astronauts are trained to experience on lift-off from earth. But of the 100 passengers aboard, only 50 sustained significant spinal cord injury.

Can these injuries be prevented? Homeowners must realize their outdoor swimming pools are a notorious hazard. Three-quarters of all spinal cord accidents occur in private pools. The most common cause is a deep dive to the bottom of the pool. Public swimming pools are three times safer, and summer camps have 12 times fewer spinal cord accidents.

Common sense can prevent a lifetime spent in a wheelchair. Don't dive into the shallow end of a pool. Don't dive off a fence around the pool. Don't dive from bridges. And never go head first into a lake until you've checked for hidden rocks. You can never learn to dive from a wheelchair. But you can dive into one with the speed of lightning.

Suppose you're a bystander when catastrophe strikes? Suspect a cord lesion immediately if the victim seems bewildered, has muscle weakness, lack of movement, numbness, or tingling sensations. What you do initially can make the difference between partial or total paralysis. Rough handling can destroy the final link between function and paralysis.

Last summer a boy struck his head on the corner of a pool. His sister, a nurse, refused to allow anyone to move him before the arrival of the ambulance. He was then transferred to the hospital on a board with traction applied to head and ankles. He remained on the stretcher board while being x-rayed. Then speedily operated on by a neurosurgeon. He made a substantial recovery.

But some cases are terrifying. One is described in the *Journal of the Royal College of Surgeons* of Edinburgh. A bush worker was hit by a tree. His companions carried him a mile through the bush, then transported him in a semi-sitting position in the back of a bus over rough road to the camp 20 miles away. The ambulance trip was another 20 miles. He was a complete paraplegic by the time he arrived at the hospital. His only chance would have been evacuation by helicopter.

Neurosurgeons suspect that improper handling by rescuers often results in further damage. One patient en route to a university hospital was diverted briefly to a small hospital for x-rays. The patient was able to move his legs on arrival at the first hospital but was totally paralyzed when he reached the second one.

This summer don't pretend that spinal cord injury can't happen in your pool. Listen to the message of the Canadian Paraplegic Association: "Play it safe. You won't be sorry."

The Perils of Waterskiing

Is it possible for a waterskier to drown while wearing a life-jacket? I always believed such precaution protected people from this fate. But last summer I witnessed a tragic accident. It should never have happened.

I had just arrived at a usually peaceful lake, but on this occasion it was a frenzy of activity. Some people were crying on the dock. Others were shouting for help. And two others were feverishly working over a prostate body, giving mouth-to-mouth resuscitation. But it was to no avail. A young, muscular, newly married man was dead. He had drowned while wearing a life-jacket. Several boats had also been in the immediate vicinity of the disaster.

What had gone wrong? All precautions seemed to have been taken. The skier was being pulled by a high-powered boat carrying two other skiers who were watching him. During one run around the lake he fell backwards, released the rope and stretched his arms up over his head. The life-jacket, which was fastened loosely, was forced by the water up over his face and trapped both arms. He would have needed to be Houdini to escape.

No one in the motorboat realized he was in trouble. When they saw something was wrong they sped back to him. But they faced another problem. The two smaller people could not pull the skier into the boat as he floundered and fought for breath. By the time other help arrived, the man was dead.

Some of the fun things in life are extremely deceptive. Everyone admits that speeding down a steep slope on skis at 60 miles an hour can be hazardous. But waterskiing looks harmless, with little or no chance of trouble. It's an impression that leads to tragedy for some families.

Dr. L.A. Pedgana, an orthopedic surgeon in Seattle, Washington, has extensive experience in waterskiing injuries. In the June 1979 issue of *Physician and Sportsmedicine* he urges doctors to play a role in preventing these accidents.

Some waterskiing injuries can have catastrophic results for young people.

For instance, Dr. Pedegana mentions five skiers who had fracture dislocations of the knee. Three of these Seattle residents lost lower legs.

How many skiing accidents occur is largely a guess. But the National Electronic Injury Surveillance System estimated that in 1976 there were 18,246 waterskiing injuries in the U.S. This estimate was based on a sampling of 119 emergency rooms that cooperated in the study.

What causes most of these injuries? The U.S. Coast Guard's computer gives a breakdown of accidents between 1971 and 1977. These figures point to the problem. Fifty-two percent of the skiers hit another boat and 12 percent struck fixed objects such as docks, pilings, and the shore. Another 5 percent collided with a floating object, and 6 percent were injured by their own boat and the propellor. Others became tangled in the rope.

This study emphasizes a vital point. Water isn't soft when it's hit at high speeds. A number of biomechanical studies have been done to determine the forces placed on legs during snow skiing. But there are no reports on the stresses on the legs while waterskiing. They must be great.

For example, none of the three skiers who lost their legs struck anything other than water. Other skiers who fell at high speeds ended up in wheelchairs due to spinal injury.

What can be done to deter similar tragedies? Don't forget that life-jackets can sometimes be a cause of injury. Some have hard material that injures the ribs. Other devices are so poorly constructed they easily fall off. And never improvise and put an adult jacket on a child. It can slip either up or down.

Be sure to have a reliable person in the back of the boat, one who can swim and is strong enough to pull an injured person into the boat. Rearview mirrors are also no substitute for an extra person in the boat. It's astounding that 21 U.S. states require either an observer or a rearview mirror! One wonders how mature legislators can pass such inadequate safety regulations.

Try to ski when there are few boats in the vicinity. Keep away from protruding docks, the shore, and swimmers. Stay clear of the propellor. A good knowledge of the lake should also prevent skiers from hitting submerged objects. And never allow young children to maneuver a high-powered boat alone.

Here's a frightening way to end a holiday. A 28-year-old woman, a petty officer in the U.S. Navy, had spent her vacation at her parents' summer cottage. A few hours before returning to the naval station she was rushed to the hospital in shock. What happened vividly illustrates one of the hazards of waterskiing. It can have life-threatening consequences.

The officer, an accomplished waterskier, lost her balance crossing the wake of another boat. She was pulled quickly from the water, but rescuers were surprised to see blood on her bathing suit. When she suddenly became weak, she was rushed to the local hospital.

Doctors soon discovered that the blood was coming from the vagina. A gauze pack was inserted to control bleeding, a blood transfusion started, and the patient prepared for immediate surgery.

Surgeons discovered a long, deep laceration extending the whole length of the vagina. A large artery spurting blood was tied off and the laceration repaired. During the procedure the patient was given three pints of blood. Postoperatively she developed a fever and continued to pass bloody urine for several days. She was able to leave the hospital on the seventh post-operative day.

What caused the injury? The officer was victim of what's called "the waterskiing douche." When she fell from her skis she struck the water with legs apart and at considerable speed. A sudden force of water had entered the vagina, rupturing the vaginal wall and injuring the urinary bladder.

How often this type of injury occurs is not known. But when searching medical literature I found several other cases had been reported. Drs. R.L. Romano and E.M. Burgess cite a case where a sudden waterskiing douche had ruptured the end of the vagina, causing peritonitis. Dr. G.F. McCarthy reported similar injuries in Australian water skiers.

Other skiers sustain injuries to the uterus and fallopian tubes complicated by pelvic abscesses. In one instance a skier became sterile due to a serious pelvic infection after the skiing douche. Female skiers have also been known to miscarry after similar accidents.

A sudden force of water can also injure males and other body cavities. Dr. Kenneth W.K. Kizer of Hawaii reports how a skiing fall in the Pacific Ocean affected a U.S. Naval diver. The following day after the fall, the diver was unable to descend to his usual depth because he could not clear his right ear. Examination revealed a bulging, deeply inflamed eardrum from water being forced into the ear's eustachian tube. He was given antibiotics and had to discontinue diving for 10 days. Other males have suffered from ruptured eardrums.

Skiers of both sexes must also guard against the waterskiing enema. Dr. D.C. Patterson, writing in *The Practitioner*, relates the story of a serious injury to the bowel. This patient had a tear that extended all the way through the bowel, causing extensive bleeding. This can occur when a skier hits the water in a sitting position or after a jump when the buttocks strike the water first.

It's usually beginning skiers wearing standard bathing suits who suffer this injury. They have not learned from competitive skiers the importance of wearing nylon-reinforced neoprene rubber skiing pants. Professionals have recommended this precautionary apparel for a long time.

5

Heart Disease, Hypertension, and Stroke

How would you like a contract with the Mafia? One that you couldn't refuse? Luckily few of us face this decision. But North Americans are often presented with another life and death contract. It's the cry of the heart, and no sensible person should ever turn it down.

Every year thousands experience the rushing pain of myocardial infarction. Fifty percent of victims don't make it to hospital. Others with chest pain are more fortunate. The heart cries out for aid long before it suddenly dies. What does this cry mean? Does it mean inevitable surgery? And can exercise soften this cry for help?

William Heberden, an English physician, first described angina pectoris (pain in the chest) in 1772. It's impossible to improve on his literary eloquence. He wrote, "There is a disorder of the breast with strong and peculiar symptoms considerable for the kind of danger belonging to it. The seat of it and the sense of strangling and anxiety with which it is attended may make it not improperly called angina pectoris."

Heberden detailed a typical attack. "They who are afflicted with it are seized while they are walking with a painful and most disagreeable sensation in the breast which seems as if it would extinguish life if it were to continue. But the moment they stand still all this uneasiness vanishes."

Another more frightening possibility was depicted by Heberden. The termination of angina pectoris is remarkable, for if the disease goes to its height the patients all suddenly fall down and perish almost immediately.

But the cause of pain and sudden death eluded doctors for nearly two centuries. In 1872 Sir Lauder Brunton, a Scottish physician, moved closer to the answer. He discovered that nitroglycerine placed under the tongue relieved chest pain. Then in 1910 Sir William Osler, a founder of Johns Hopkins Medical School, made a prediction. He speculated that the heart's coronary vessels went into spasm.

Osler couldn't prove his theory before the invention of the electrocardiogram (EKG). This machine eventually revealed that angina pectoris resulted from an abnormal pattern of electrical waves from the heart. Cardiologists refer to this change as "a depression of the ST segment."

A heart that cries for help is like a faltering gasoline pump. The pump motor needs an adequate supply of gasoline and a good exhaust system. Similarly the heart's muscle needs a flow of blood. Starved of oxygen-laden blood, the cardiac muscle develops pain. A decreased blood flow also permits waste products of metabolism to build up in the cardiac muscle, irritating the nerves and adding to the pain.

But there's some good news for these patients. The chest discomfort acts like a fire detector that warns of smoke before a blaze erupts. The pain is often so severe that patients must stop whatever they're doing. This sudden inactivity allows the blood flow to build up oxygen in the heart and saves the person's life.

Nature's warning alarm tells doctors that the heart has developed rusty plumbing. A faulty lifestyle, general aging, or poor heredity has produced atherosclerosis of the coronary vessels. And it's vitally important at this point for doctors to assess the extent of this biological rust.

How is it done? First an EKG is taken while the patient is resting. Later another is taken while the patient exercises on a treadmill. Doctors gradually increase the amount of exercise until the person develops chest pain, or other symptoms say it's time to stop the test.

This test provides physicians with a revealing clue. If angina is triggered by minimal exertion, arterial rust is severe. The warning may be the lull before the storm of myocardial infarction. But if it takes strenuous exercise to recreate chest pain the outlook is better.

Cardiologists use angiography when chest pain is produced by minimal exercise. A tiny plastic tube is introduced through an artery in either the arm or leg. This catheter is gradually pushed towards coronary vessels and x-ray movies pinpoint any obstruction.

The location of the cry for help is important. For example, a major obstruction of the left coronary artery may cause sudden death. A coronary bypass operation might be necessary to prevent this calamity.

Not all people with angina need surgery. X-rays sometimes show that nature produces extra vessels to circumvent the obstruction. A graduated exercise program can then help the heart so it need not cry out so desperately.

When Is Chest Pain Not Due to Heart Disease?

"In the night imagining some fear, how easy is a bush supposed a bear." William Shakespeare's words are as true today as they were 500 years ago. Ninety-nine percent of North Americans who suddenly develop chest pain conclude immediately it's due to a heart problem. But in many instances the cause of the pain is somewhere else. It may even be Texidor's twinge.

Recently I saw an apprehensive 50-year-old woman who was convinced she had angina. She described the pain as a burning sensation deep in the center of the chest. But she also complained of a sour taste in the back of her mouth.

This suggested she had an inflammation of the foodpipe (esophagitis), which occurs when the stomach's acid regurgitates into the lower end of the esophagus. She was given an antacid and in a couple of weeks the discomfort had disappeared.

In one research study doctors did extensive examinations on 100 consecutive patients seen in the emergency department complaining of chest pain. Of these only 51 were suffering from coronary heart disease. Others had a variety of problems such as stomach ulcer, gallstones, inflammation of the pancreas, muscular pain due to trauma, or just gas in the large bowel.

Some patients with chest pain suffer from the slipping rib syndrome. This occurs when the cartilage of the tenth rib becomes dislocated and overrides the cartilage of the ninth rib. Sharp pain then occurs when the body is in a peculiar posture. The pain can be reproduced by hooking the fingers under the lower rib cage and tugging firmly towards the patient's shoulder. This maneuver may also elicit a clicking noise.

A hypersensitive xiphoid process, the knob at the bottom of the breast bone, may be the culprit. This is very distressing to patients, because it causes substernal pain in the same location as coronary pain. This discomfort can also be reproduced by pushing on the xiphoid process.

Tietze's syndrome is often a cause of undiagnosed chest pain. This is a localized swelling of a single costochrondral junction, the point where the ribs attach to the sternum. It generally results in a constant aching sensation, but sharp pains can be present. This diagnosis is made by pushing on the costochrondral junction, which triggers the pain.

Some patients with bronchospasm become apprehensive that tightness in their chest is due to heart disease, but the wheezing and coughing point to the cause of the pain. Pleuritic pain can also cause needless worry about the heart. This pain is usually associated with pneumonia or a blood clot in the lung, or it may be the result of Bornholm's disease, often called the "devil's grip." This illness is due to coxsakievirus B, and usually occurs in the summer or fall. The onset is acute, with headache, fever, and productive cough and chest pain.

Uptight patients are especially prone to complain of "fluttery" pains in the chest. These are usually heart palpitations which are perceived as pain. The clue to diagnosis is that the pain always coincides with the heartbeat.

Herpes is a common cause of chest pain, particularly in older people. Prior to the eruption of the vesicular lesions, the virus causes a burning, tingling pain in the chest, usually localized to one or two ribs.

Most people have never heard of Texidor's twinge. But nearly everyone has experienced this pain at some time. It's also referred to as "a precordial catch." The setting usually provides the clue to the diagnosis. The pain occurs while the person is sitting, and is a sharp sudden pain usually in the left chest. It is eased by shallow breathing or a change in position and lasts just a few moments. Texidor's twinge is believed to be due to a transient pinching of the pleura lining the chest wall or a pinching of the heart's pericardium. It is more likely to happen in thin people.

If you have chest pain, consult your doctor. But remember there's a good chance it's the bush and not the bear.

Plan Early to Prevent Premature Heart Attack

Fifty percent of heart attack victims don't get a second chance. One minute they're feeling fine. The next moment sudden death is their first and last symptom. Is this appointment with death inevitable? Or can change in lifestyle circumvent some catastrophes in the prime of life?

Most people who are destined for heart attack face one formidable obstacle. They either don't know or ignore the fact that the conditions leading to arthereosclerosis (hardening of the arteries) and a premature coronary start early in life. Moreover, it's not just a single bad habit that clogs the artery. It's a series of poor practices that finally pulls the trigger.

How can parents help keep themselves and their children from an early demise? The establishment of a sound lifestyle as soon as possible is still at the top of the preventive list. But how can we expect children to develop sane dietary habits if we are fat and flatulent at 40? Or replace milk with soft drinks? Or continue to consume pack after pack of cigarettes? Or depend on the turning of the TV knob as our main form of exercise? A faulty living style is almost always a family affair.

It's also a mistake to concentrate primarily on the "maybes" of heart disease. Ten years from now many of these theories may be proven wrong. In the meantime millions of North Americans ignore the main killer, about which there is no debate. Obesity is still the biggest culprit in heart disease. It also sets the stage for a number of other problems.

Excess weight is a prime cause of hypertension. This in turn increases the chance of stroke, heart failure, and eye and kidney disease. Never make the mistake of categorizing disease into neat, isolated packages. If a car pulls too much weight, many parts start to break down.

What is the best way for families to avoid an atherogenic way of life? I think it makes sense to aim towards a lower-fat diet. It may help to lower the blood cholesterol and lessen the chance of atheromatous plaque forming in the coronary vessels. There's no 100 percent proof that it works. But if doctors waited for total proof on most treatments they would end up advising next to nothing.

There are some convincing animal experiments which link a high-cholesterol diet to hardening of the arteries. It's also wise to consider what happened when the U.S. occupied the Pacific islands. The islanders became more affluent and changed their old dietary habits. They developed a taste for junk foods. They littered the beaches with beer cans. They became soft and sedentary. Now degenerative conditions such as heart disease and diabetes are a number one problem.

Suppose the cholesterol theory is wrong. Going easy on fats won't have been a complete loss. Fats contain twice as many calories as proteins and carbohydrates. It's one way to lose pounds. And there's little doubt that obese people generally have more atherosclerosis than thin ones.

The family should also put some action into life. Modern technology has made too many of us motionless sloths. Paul Dudley White, Harvard's famous heart specialist, aptly summed up the problem. He said, "When I graduated from medical school in 1911, I had never heard of coronary thrombosis which is one of the chief threats to life in Canada and the U.S. today. What an astonishing development in one's own lifetime!" Dudley White also practiced what he preached. Late in life he still rode a bicycle every day. He was convinced that exercise started early in life helped to maintain a healthy heart.

I don't think it's necessary to give up all the pleasures in life. Moderate drinking does not appear to increase coronary disease. But young people who throw away the cigarettes have a longer life expectancy than those who continue to smoke.

Remember that keeping away from coronary attack is really a pediatric problem, not an adult one. Discard your bad habits at an early age. Postpone living dangerously until you're 80. The worst that a bottle of Scotch a day can do at that age is kill you.

Remember, too, that nothing you do will ever confer immortality. Sooner or later in old age something will claim you. The real challenge of the game is not to depart in the early innings.

Stress and Your Heart

My red-headed Irish friend was built like the boxing champion John L. Sullivan. He was tired after a long day in surgery, but we were looking forward to a hockey game at the Boston Garden on a stormy, snowy night. As we drove through the city, the light at one intersection turned green, but my weary colleague was slow stepping on the gas. The result was a sudden loud honk from the car behind us. Immediately the Irish temper flared. My friend jumped out, walked back to the car behind, opened the door, grabbed the keys out of the lock and with a mighty toss threw them into a snowbank. I'll never know whether the driver found his keys. We drove on our way. But I'm sure he'll think twice before he uses his horn on a snowy night.

Dr. Meyer Friedman and Dr. Ray Rosenman would have something to say about this scenario. These two U.S. researchers in psychology would quickly classify my Irish friend as a type A personality. The same label would probably apply to the car-honking Bostonian behind us. And they might predict an early coronary for both.

These American doctors believe that people can be classified into two different personality types. Type A are workaholics, perfectionists, and overachievers who want to set the world on fire. The more relaxed type B personalities are less likely to succumb to fatal coronary attack.

As an example Peter Finch, the actor, had just finished making the movie *Network*. His schedule had been grueling and the film emotionally draining. He faced a round of TV and press appearances. A major effort was mounted to keep him in the public eye before the Academy Award winners were announced. He died suddenly in the lobby of the Beverly Hills Hotel while waiting to appear on *Good Morning America*.

Consider the Nixon family! The wife of the former President suffered a stroke on July 8, 1976. An unconfirmed report suggested she was stricken while reading a best-selling book that attacked her husband. The President also encountered phlebitis at the same time, an ailment that is sometimes suspected of being stress-related.

Were these problems just coincidence? Some researchers would say no. They point to Japanese-Americans. Those in San Francisco who follow traditional ways and customs have the same low incidence of myocardial infarction as their countrymen in Japan. Those who become "Americanized" have two to five times the amount of heart disease.

The *Journal of the American Medical Association* added more evidence in 1975. It reported a study of 3,000 males between the ages of 39 and 59. The men who were competitive and aggressive and always hurrying had twice the rate of coronary attack of the more relaxed individuals.

How do you know if you're type A? Dr. James C. Paupst of Toronto suggests ways of classifying yourself. For example, do you always ask for the restaurant bill before you're finished eating dinner? Do you hurry slow speakers? Do you rush through lovemaking? Do you get many speeding tickets? And are you a constant toe-tapper?

If so, can you change your ways? Dr. Hans Selye of Montreal, an authority on stress, believed that everyone can smooth rough spots off their psyche. It's reasonable to strive for improvement, but never reach for perfection. Keep in mind the pleasant aspects of life and don't dwell on the ugly. If you suffer a major defeat, don't become frustrated. Instead remember past achievements. And accept the fact that men are not created equal. If you're not a leader of men, don't get a coronary trying to be one.

Drs. Friedman and Rosenman suggest other ways of liberating yourself. Don't think of more than one thing at a time. It's said that even Einstein, when he tied his shoelaces, just thought about the bow. Then when you're uptight about a problem, ask yourself if it will have any importance in five years' time. And patronize restaurants where you know the service is slow. If you can't find anything to say to your wife while waiting for the soup, you need another companion.

Dr. Paupst says we should all get rid of the hurry sickness. Don't try to finish everything by the end of the day. As one wise sage once remarked, "Only a corpse is completely finished." He pleads with people to stop rushing around, stop over-committing themselves and to eliminate deadlines.

I like to believe he's wrong. I'd prefer to think one drops from a coronary because of obesity, hypertension, smoking, and genetic background. Yet I admit to a lingering doubt. Dr. Paupst may be right, so why take a chance? I'm reading how his method will change me into a type B personality. I haven't raced through a yellow light for over a week. Who knows, he may even convince me to give up deadlines.

Heart Disease Isn't What It Used to Be

Oscar Wilde once wrote, "The advantage of emotions is that they lead us astray." But in 1891 Wilde wasn't aware that the emotions had any effect on the coronary arteries. Nor that doctors would revise their theories of anginal pain. Heart disease today isn't what it used to be. And there's evidence that doctors should refer their patients with angina to psychiatrists.

Doctors used to be convinced that anginal pain and coronary heart attacks were due to artherosclerosis. The hardening and gradual plugging of blood vessels reduces the supply of blood to the heart's muscle. The result is recurrent attacks of angina when the heart is forced to work harder with exercise. And it can end with the crushing pain of a myocardial infarction.

But unanswered questions remained. For instance, why do heart attacks occur in people who do not have fat-blocked coronary arteries? And why do some patients have anginal pain at rest, but not during exertion? Physicians suspect it might be the result of coronary spasm. But how could they prove it? Autopsy often fails to reveal a blood clot in the coronary vessels. But there's no way of proving the arteries went into spasm at the time of death.

In 1959 Myron Prinzmetal of Los Angeles suggested that this did indeed occur. He studied a group of patients whose coronary vessels had narrowed only slightly and who complained of angina only at rest or during sleep. Their electrocardiograms (EKGs) were significant; the tracings showed the exact opposite of patients who suffered anginal pain with exertion due to severe narrowing of atherosclerotic vessels. But both types of patients were relieved of pain by nitroglycerine tablets.

Dr. Prinzmetal deduced that spasm triggered the pain in those with only slightly narrowed vessels. But the majority of physicians were skeptical of his theory.

As new techniques were developed for studying the heart, evidence accumulated that confirmed Dr. Prinzmetal's theory. For instance, an investigator was taking x-rays of the coronary arteries when the patient suddenly complained of chest pain. At that precise moment the x-rays revealed total obstruction of the coronary vessels.

Dr. Albert A. Kattus, chief of cardiology at the University of California, provided more evidence. During a coronary bypass operation the patient's blood pressure suddenly fell, the heartbeat weakened, and the heart began to dilate. Then the coronary vessel that was to receive the graft went into spasm, closing completely and blocking the flow of blood. Equally important, the EKG findings were identical with those observed during bouts of nocturnal anginal pain.

Dr. Attilio Maseri of Hammersmith Hospital, London, England, says spasm accounts for 20 percent of anginal pain. Others, like Dr. John S. Schroeder of Stanford University, believe this is just the tip of the iceberg. He thinks spasm plays a role in nearly all cases.

This research shouldn't come as a surprise. Dr. Peter Reich, head of psychiatry at the Brigham and Women's Hospital in Boston, studied patients who had experienced life-threatening rhythmic disorders of the heart. In one case out of five he found major and unusual emotional distress occurred within 24 hours of the attack. Since this can happen, why shouldn't lesser degrees of emotional tension trigger angina?

Can spasm be prevented? Researchers claim that the ultimate cause of spasm is the entry of calcium ions into the arterial wall. A new group of drugs called "calcium antagonists" are now available to counteract this chemical reaction. They may also help to curb the increasing number of coronary bypass operations.

I think that patients with angina should hear a strong, clear message from this research. There is still no way to remove artherosclerosis from a blocked coronary artery. But if a spasm is a contributing factor in anginal pain for the first time, part of the cure lies in your own hands. Like patients with stomach ulcers or tension headaches, it's time to reassess your lifestyle.

Some patients with spasm angina may need the help of a psychiatrist. But I think that most just need the ear of a sympathetic family doctor who understands the patient's job, wife, and personality as well as his heart. He can't change the spots on a leopard. But he may be able to pinpoint and correct emotional situations that tie your coronary arteries into a dangerous knot.

Salt and Hypertension

Doctors should tell people the truth about hypertension. They keep saying they don't know the cause of high blood pressure, then prescribe a variety of questionable drugs in an attempt to lower the pressure. But history and animals have shown for years that excessive consumption of salt is a major cause. Yet in an age of mind-boggling computers and instant communication, this message is not reaching medical consumers.

Scientists first speculated in 1904 that salt was the villain in this disease. Since that time they've been amassing evidence by comparing people who traditionally eat a large amount of salt and those who do not.

Dr. Lot B. Page, Professor of Medicine at Tufts University in Boston, has traveled to the far corners of the world to study this problem. His conclusion? There are at least 20 national populations where the blood pressure does not increase with age. They include Greenland Eskimos, Congo Pygmies, Cook

Islanders, Kalahari Bushmen, Yanomamo Indians of Brazil, Melanesians, Polynesians, Australian Aborigines, Africans, and Chinese.

The diets of these people vary widely. Polynesians consume coconuts and fish. The Kalahari Bushmen survive on berries, insects, and game. The Eskimos at one time were almost wholly carnivorous. The Melanesians live on root crops. And these people live in such diverse regions as the Arctic and the desert.

Why are these groups free of hypertension? Scientists once believed it was because they had developed over the centuries a genetic resistance to hypertension. But this theory was proven wrong. It became apparent that these people also became hypertensive when they developed Western habits or moved to Western countries.

Salt is the crucial factor, far outweighing factors such as stress, crowding, a sedentary lifestyle, or obesity. For instance a study in 1976 of the nomads of Iran, primitive sheepherders, showed that 15 percent had hypertension. They're thin and active but addicted to salty foods.

A research team from Harvard University also investigated tribes on the Solomon Islands. The Lau fishermen who boiled their food in sea water had a higher rate of hypertension than neighboring tribes which cooked with fresh water.

Veterinarians know that hypertension is a human disease. Animals are normally free of this problem. But the late Lewis K. Dahl of Brookhaven National Laboratory in New York added large amounts of salt to a colony of rats. They, too, developed high blood pressure.

Salt is sodium chloride and sodium is the culprit. The human body needs just 200 mg of sodium a day. North Americans consume an average of 12,000 mg a day. Excess salt retains water, causing bodily tissues to expand, squeezing blood vessels, and increasing blood pressure.

How do we get so much sodium? Much of it is due to commercially prepared foods whose contents are unlisted or disguised so that the consumer is unaware. For instance, frozen peas contain 100 times as much sodium as fresh peas. Canned peas contain 200 times as much of this ingredient. And one popular fast food hamburger contains 500 mg of sodium.

There's another trap. Many salted foods do not taste salty. For instance, two slices of white bread contain more sodium than an ounce of salty potato chips, an ounce of corn flakes twice as much sodium as an ounce of salted peanuts. And sometimes you exchange one devil for another. Synthetic sweeteners used by people to avoid sugar contain sodium.

Life is full of inconsistencies. Our government spends huge sums of money to treat complications of hypertension, the bursting blood vessels that cause stroke, or hearts, kidneys and eyes that gradually fail because of increased pressure. Yet we allow manufacturers who care nothing about the health of the nation to pour tons of salt into packaged foods.

How can the consumer protect his health from the ravages of salt? A good start is to remove the salt shaker from the table. Tell the cook to go easy on salt in cooking. And avoid salted peanuts, pretzels, and potato chips.

Make an effort to become aware of the sodium content of common foods. For example, a 3½ ounce serving of pretzels contains 7,800 mg of sodium. Dill pickles contain 4,000 mg, regular soy sauce 6,082 mg, green olives 2,400 mg, processed cheese 1,421 mg, and Canadian bacon 2,555 mg. Try to avoid products that list salt or sodium-containing additives near the top of the ingredients list. And remember that canned soup and soup powders, often contain over 1,000 mg of sodium.

I've often told readers to trust the farmer and beware of the manufacturers of packaged foods. Fresh corn contains 1 mg of sodium, a cup of canned corn 384 mg. Three ounces of fresh shrimp contain only 137 mg; the same amount of canned shrimp has 1,955 mg. Need I say more?

How to Lower Blood Pressure Without Drugs

The figures are staggering. It's estimated that 35 million people in Canada and the U.S. have high blood pressure. An additional 25 million have borderline hypertension. Like too much pressure in a tire, this triggers a variety of blow-outs in the human body. Some people succumb to strokes, others to kidney and heart failure or blindness. But to treat this tragic disorder it's not always necessary to reach for drugs. More and more evidence indicates that changes in lifestyle can help to stop the constant pounding of the body's organs.

There are several options available. The overweight person with hypertension is lucky in at least one aspect. Unlike the thin person with high blood pressure, he has the opportunity to reduce; weight loss alone can sometimes return blood pressure to normal. Moreover, it's not always necessary to trim weight to the desired listing in the insurance tables. Just losing half the weight can produce a drop in pressure.

At the same time increased physical activity will help—climbing stairs rather than using elevators, for instance. But the most efficient way to lower pressure is by aerobic exercises. This involves sustained activity that continues for 30 minutes three or four times a week. Swimming, skipping rope, jogging, bicycling, or fast walking are all excellent aerobic exercises.

Doctors in the past have cast a skeptical eye on the role of exercise in lowering pressure. Several studies were unable to separate the effects of exercise on blood pressure from those of weight loss, salt restriction, and stress reduction. Now there is decreasing pessimism about the effect of exercise in fighting hypertension.

Dr. John Martin of the Veterans Administration Hospital in Jackson, Mississippi, has carried out extensive studies on aerobic exercise. He believes sustained exercise lowers hypertension by reducing psychological stress. He's convinced that stress impairs the body's ability to regulate fluid and salt balance.

Dr. Norman Kaplan of Dallas, a noted expert on hypertension, says the evidence that aerobic exercise lowers blood pressure grows stronger every day. In his words, "I'm willing to believe it, but we need more hard evidence."

How much aerobic exercise lowers blood pressure varies from patient to patient. Some patients were able to stop taking their medication. Others sustained a 10 to 20 percent drop in pressure. The best results were seen in patients who had never taken any drugs for hypertension and in those people who had an overactive nervous system. But to get results patients had to use 70 to 80 percent of the heart's pumping capacity during exercise.

Eliminating the use of cigarettes also fights hypertension. Smoking packs a double whammy. It worsens the risk of cardiovascular complications for any degree of hypertension. In addition, the nicotine in a single cigarette can increase the pressure by 10 points, with the effect lasting 15 minutes. For the average smoker that amounts to eight hours of nicotine hypertension a day.

It's also helpful to decrease caffeine intake. We know that the caffeine in two to three cups of coffee raises the blood pressure 10 to 14 points. In one study patients with hypertension were asked to abstain from smoking and coffee overnight. The result? The pressure dropped from 13 to 20 points.

Should you give up having an alcoholic drink before dinner? Studies show that one martini has no consistent effect on blood pressure. But high blood pressure is seen more often in those who consume more than three alcoholic drinks a day.

Beware of over-the-counter medications to treat asthma, or cold, allergy, and appetite-suppressant drugs, which have the potential to increase blood pressure. Phenylpropanolamine and caffeine are often present in these preparations. And go easy on salt. About 33 percent of patients with mild hypertension can return the pressure to normal levels by a low salt diet.

Avoiding high blood pressure is worth a change in lifestyle. The payoff is a longer life and less chance of a stroke and heart attack. As well, a simple improvement in lifestyle carries no adverse side effects.

Calcium and Hypertension

Dr. David McCarron, a hypertension specialist at the University of Oregon, claims researchers have made a major error. For years they've assumed hypertension was caused by an excess of something, particularly salt. But it now appears that a lack of calcium sets the stage for this major killer. He presents some interesting evidence.

In one study 170 patients with hypertension were given 100 mg of calcium a day for eight weeks. Forty-five percent of these patients were cured of hypertension.

The National Center for Health Statistics carried out another study on 21,000 Americans to analyze their eating habits. The survey failed to show any consistent relationship between salt and hypertension, but it showed a strong correlation between dietary calcium intake and high blood pressure. Hypertensives consumed 18 percent less calcium than those with normal pressure.

In another study Johns Hopkins medical students were asked to eat an extra 1,000 mg of calcium a day for 20 weeks. The students all had normal pressures at the start of the study. But at the end of 20 weeks the blood pressure of the male students had dropped by 10 percent. The pressure of . female students decreased by 8 percent.

It's also worthwhile noting that black Americans have a higher incidence of hypertension than the rest of the population. They are also known to have a reduced intake of dietary calcium.

Post-menopausal women we know are plagued by osteoporosis, a condition in which their bones become thin and brittle. It's a major cause of fractured hips in the elderly. Several studies indicate that a lack of calcium is a primary cause of this problem. Calcium-deficient women are also more likely to suffer from hypertension than women of the same age without osteoporosis.

Calcium isn't the only factor associated with hypertension. A U.S. government study revealed that the greater the intake of calcium, potassium, phosphorus, and magnesium, the lower the blood pressure.

Dr. McCarron says that salt restriction will lower blood pressure in just 5 percent of hypertensive patients. He adds that many hypertensives actually have a low intake of salt in the first place. Does this mean that salt is out and calcium in? McCarron admits that about 30 to 40 percent of hypertensives are salt sensitive. But unless patients have this problem, he sees no reason why they should follow a salt-restricted diet.

One fact in McCarron's report is of particular interest. A survey was carried out on 2,000 Southern Californians to see if their consumption of cholesterol was related to heart disease. Much to their surprise they discovered that the more dairy products were consumed, the lower the blood pressure. They concluded that a balanced diet containing both cholesterol and calcium in moderate amounts helps to protect against high blood pressure. This finding should ring a loud, clear bell.

For years I've told readers that blaming dairy products for heart attacks is like blaming the iceberg for sinking the *Titanic*. I've also cautioned that obesity and hypertension often go together. Now McCarron believes that lean people generally have a high intake of calcium. Obese people are often found to have a deficiency of calcium, which is why the blood pressure skyrockets.

It's important to keep an open mind on medical issues, but not so open your brains fall out. So let's not get carried away in believing that calcium is the be all and end all to cure this life-threatening disease.

The smart medical consumer will still toss the salt shaker off the table. He'll stay thin and active. He will eat a balanced diet. And he won't totally blame hens and cows for the epidemic of degenerative disease that is sweeping North America. Rather, he'll place the blame where it belongs—on a way of life that is generally careless, self-indulgent, and immoderate.

Is It Too Late to Butt Out After a Heart Attack?

What should smokers do after they've suffered a heart attack? Does it make sense to butt out at this stage? Is it too late in the game to change a faulty lifestyle? These are pertinent questions when the cool hand of death touches the shoulder.

Dr. Dr. Claes Wilhelmsson, professor at the University of Gotenborg, Sweden, followed 3,303 heart attack victims under 65 years of age for $10\frac{1}{2}$ years. Of this group 1,020 were smokers, and 55 percent decided to stop the habit.

The result should open the eyes of anyone who has felt the crushing pain of myocardial infarction. Dr. Wilhelmsson found that those who quit smoking had half the death rate of those who refused to stop. His advice to doctors? The most important thing a physician can do is to convince heart attack patients to stop smoking.

His results showed that eight years after a coronary, 74 percent of the former smokers were living, but only 55 percent of the continuing smokers. For patients under 50 years of age the outcome following cessation of smoking was even better.

There was another big plus for former smokers. They also suffered fewer non-fatal recurrences. For example, the non-fatal reinfarction rate for this group was 21 percent. But for smokers the frequency jumped to 38 percent.

But how did Dr. Wilhelmsson convince 55 percent of his patients to butt out? He said the whole secret was timing. He found it was almost impossible to persuade patients to throw away cigarettes once they left the hospital. The only hope was to counsel coronary victims "when the brush with death was still vivid in their memory."

The professor stressed that he doesn't have a magic message for smokers. He believes the time for fairy tales is over once a coronary strikes. So he tells patients the truth. That he's eager to help them. That it's never too late to quit. That it is really the only thing the patient can do to help himself.

Fifty-five percent is a good batting average. But why were 45 percent of Swedes crazy enough to continue smoking after a coronary? And an even greater number of North Americans?

Is there a way to convince people to butt out before a heart attack? Dr. Walter Rosser, professor of family medicine at Ottawa University, believes we're not using enough posters to drive home the hazards of smoking. He also advocates placing a red sticker on the medical charts of all smokers. It would demonstrate vividly that doctors consider them a special health risk.

Dr. Michael Russel of the Maudley Hospital in London, England, believes nicotine gum helps patients over the hurdle. He reports curing 65 percent with this method. Only 20 percent of non-gum smokers kicked the habit.

Butting out is like telling a dog to stop chasing its tail. Every puff on a cigarette sends nicotine to the brain in a few seconds. It increases the blood pressure and heart rate. And smokers start to chase their tails.

Momentarily smokers feel more relaxed and are able to concentrate better. But when the level of nicotine in the blood falls, withdrawal symptoms make them reach for another cigarette.

Will low-nicotine cigarettes mean more butting out? One experiment revealed that when smokers made this switch they had to catch up the loss of nicotine in other ways. Some, without realizing it, smoked more cigarettes than usual. Others left smaller butts in the ashtray, inhaled more deeply, or held the smoke in the lungs longer.

I think there is only one way to butt out. Cutting off a dog's tail bit by bit hurts more. Humans react the same way to piecemeal measures. The gradual loss of lungs from bronchiectasis or emphysema or the increased risk of malignancy commands an immediate stop to suicidal tail-chasing.

Regrettably many North Americans will continue to succumb to preventable lung disease and heart attacks. They are much like pregnant teenagers who believe "it won't happen" to them. But lives could be saved if both government and doctors shed their cloaks of hypocrisy.

Isn't it ironic that the government spends billions to treat what has been labeled "smokepox" by Professor George Lewis at McMaster University, yet it refuses to ban smoking in hospitals. It's equally shocking that some U.S. hospitals attempted to ban smoking in hospitals but lost the battle. Why? Because their medical staffs refused unqualified support to the ban on smokepox.

Much Ado About the "Clicky" Heart Valve

Here's a plea to doctors: Let's stop scaring patients half to death with casual comments about their "clicky" heart valves. We might admit to ourselves instead that we've discovered a new heart sound. Evidence now indicates the the noise of the heart isn't important, that we're causing needless worry by informing patients of a "mitral valve prolapse." Patients who've been given this diagnosis write anxious letters to me, convinced they're destined for an early demise, and repeatedly ask if surgery can correct the problem.

Doctors usually refer to this medical finding as a "mitral click." For years physicians have been aware of the clicking sound of some hearts. But in the past they didn't get too excited about it for two reasons. First, such patients often appear to be healthy. Second, they believed the click originated beyond the heart, somewhere else in the chest cavity.

But progress is sometimes a mixed blessing. Researchers developed new listening devices such as the phonocardiogram and echocardiogram. These machines have proven the mitral click is due to a floppy mitral heart valve. The mitral valve separates two main chambers of the heart. A floppy mitral valve is like the swing door of a western saloon; its hinges are a little too long, allowing the valve to swing back slightly into one chamber of the heart when blood is forced through., The result is a heart click.

Doctors don't agree on how many people have this disorder. In one research study 107 medical workers were examined with a stethoscope and 10 percent had a heart click. When this same group was examined with a phonocardiogram the incidence increased to 17 percent. With the echocardiogram it jumped to 21 percent.

Who has a click and who hasn't also depends on the experience of the doctor. The click can be missed if a patient is examined in just one position. Also, this noise comes and goes. If a patient is examined on just one occasion, there may be no sound.

Why did doctors become concerned about the mitral click? Some patients with with mitral prolapse have complained of chest pain, heart palpitations, shortness of breath, and fatigue. But often these symptoms didn't appear until after the patient was told about the click. This shouldn't surprise anyone. We know some patients become "cardiac cripples" if they're told of an unimportant heart murmur. The diagnosis, mitral valve prolapse, sounds even more ominous.

At one time there were also isolated reports of sudden death in patients with this diagnosis. Now we know that these people had other serious heart problems that caused their premature demise.

Doctors once believed another theory—that floppy valves were prone to develop small blood clots on them. These might travel to the brain, causing some patients to die of stroke. But attempts to find the source of these clots on clicky valves has been a dismal failure.

So don't start preparing your will if someone informs you of a mitral click. The human body isn't perfect, and it has an amazing capacity to adjust to imperfection. It's hard to believe, however, that one in five of us has a mitral valve deficiency. And if so, it can hardly be called a disease.

Dr. Ernest Fallen, chief of cardiology at McMaster University, has reassuring news. In 294 consecutive autopsies the floppy valve was seen in only 5 percent of cases, and not one in the under-40 age group. Dr. Fallen suggests facetiously that many people with the click must be immortal. Or that they never have an autopsy. Or that the problem miraculously disappears prior to death.

There's only one logical conclusion. The click is due to a slight variation in the architecture of the valve. This causes a slight difference in valve function.

Dr. Fallen suggests that doctors should reassure the patient if a mitral click is heard. I have another suggestion. Listen to this interesting sound. Make a note of it on the patient's chart. But, please, don't tell the patient. Otherwise you might as well tell him that his crooked legs or deviated nasal septum will shorten his life.

Watch Out for Signs of the Little Stroke

Most people associate strokes with an aging parent or relative. This is a dangerous misconception. One third of all stroke victims are under 55 years of age, and two thirds are below 65. During 1978 Montreal can expect 4,000 new cases. Regina will need beds for about 300 stroke patients. And cities with populations of 25,000 will have 50 victims admitted to their hospitals. This year 50,000 Canadians will either die or become chronically disabled from this disease. But amid all the gloom there's a bit of good news. Some strokes can be detected before they strike. Some can even be prevented.

The human brain was created with one shortcoming. For instance, a coronary patient may fully recover from his mishap. Heart muscle can repair itself to a degree depending on the extent of injury. So can an alcoholic liver. But stroke victims don't have this advantage. Brain tissue has no reparative power. A major stroke normally leaves a defect. Some patients experience loss of muscle control, others a personality change or an inability to think coherently. There's all the more reason to try to prevent a big stroke.

Some strokes have no warning signs. In 25 percent of cases a blood vessel suddenly ruptures in the brain. The other 75 percent of strokes develop when an artery becomes blocked, shutting off the supply of oxygen to the brain. Patients in this latter group are often warned by a minor storm before the tornado hits.

Doctors refer to these early warnings as transient ischemic attacks or TIAs. They result when there is a sudden temporary decrease in the blood supply to one part of the brain. Often the cause is a small blood clot that breaks off the wall of an atheromatous plaque (a form of arteriosclerosis in which yellowish plaques containing fat and cholesterol narrow the artery). This tiny clot is carried by the bloodstream and lodges in the brain. It can be the prelude to a major stroke.

The most dramatic symptom is sudden blindness in one eye. Sometimes it involves the entire vision of the eye. Other patients will notice a dark curtain descending or ascending over half of the visual field. It takes only 10 to 15 seconds to develop and the duration of blindness is just as brief.

More commonly patients complain of repeated dizzy spells or a sudden fall due to numbness of the legs. Others experience numbness of the tongue or mouth. Still others suffer paralysis or numbness of one side of the body.

There is some reassuring news from one extensive study of patients with TIAs. It shows a tendency for these attacks to cease in 50 percent of cases in one to three years. But there is no way of knowing who will improve and who will have a major attack.

You can start early in life to prevent a small or a large stroke. The handwriting of future trouble is clearly on the wall for some people. They become obese early in life, inactive, and develop hypertension. Like an over-inflated tire, they suffer a blowout, in the brain.

Don't forget that obesity is the central problem of many diseases. For instance, weight causing too much pressure on the pancreas instigates diabetes. This in turn results in premature aging of other arteries. Atheromatous plaques form within arterial walls and set the stage for stroke. Other factors, such as cigarette smoking and too much cholesterol, also seem to play a role.

But if you've unwittingly done all the wrong things and have suffered a TIA, is there anything that can be done to ward off the big stroke?

Doctors have attacked this problem from two standpoints in the past. They have tried to reverse the atheromatous process and thereby increase the flow of blood to the brain. But dredging a blocked artery isn't as easy as removing sludge from a polluted river. So far there's no good evidence that once formed an atheromatous plaque can be made to shrink.

Doctors had another idea. Why not attack blood in the same way as obesity? Fat people have to slim down to crawl through a small window. So why not thin the blood so it can more easily squeeze past a constricted artery?

The theory makes sense. But there have been a few problems. Sometimes anticoagulants thin the blood too much, causing bleeding into the brain and other organs. Patients on a routine of anticoagulants also seem to have the same death rate as those who receive nothing.

Young People Should Listen to Pogo's Advice

Why does a doctor suddenly move his stethoscope from the heart to the neck? Has he had a bad night, or forgotten his anatomy? Can this examination prevent a crippling stroke? And what can teenagers learn from Pogo's advice?

The statistics on strokes are staggering. During the next 24 hours 1,200 North Americans will suffer the trauma of a stroke. And of the 400,000 victims who experience this cerebrovascular accident this year, 200,000 will die. The rest are often left with disabilities worse than death.

Some strokes, similar to the blowout of a tire, result from sudden rupture of a blood vessel in the brain. But the majority of cerebrovascular accidents are caused by blockage of the internal carotid artery. An atheromatous plaque has shut off the blood supply to the brain.

The carotid artery is particularly prone to the development of athero-sclerosis. The common carotid splits into two branches, the external branch delivering blood to the face and scalp, the internal carrying blood to the brain. At the point where the artery divides, the flow of blood increases in velocity. This creates a suction effect and over a period of years causes wear and tear to the endothelial lining of the blood vessel. It's believed such damage is one factor stimulating the development of atherosclerosis.

Partial obstruction of the internal carotid artery results in what doctors refer to as a "bruit" or murmur. The constricted artery causes a decrease in the blood flow. But as in a stream that suddenly narrows, currents and eddys are produced just beyond the constricted area. These currents cause the sound of a neck murmur heard through the doctor's stethoscope.

A carotid bruit can usually be heard when about half of the artery is blocked by antheromatous plaque. In the past physicians have not agreed about its significance. Now doctors know this often indicates an impending problem.

Dr. John L. Ochsner is professor of surgery at Tulane University in New Orleans. He says that about 60 percent of these fatty lesions increase in size over a 10-year period.

There's other ominous news. Patients with a bruit may be free of symptoms but 47 percent still develop either small or large strokes during a 10-year interval. If symptoms do accompany the bruit, there's a 10 times greater chance of a major cerebrovascular accident.

Carotid arteries with a large blockage require an operation to clean out the plaque and prevent a major stroke. In less severe cases an aspirin a day can keep the blood from forming a clot on the atheromatous plaque.

How can you fight atherosclerosis and the start of carotid bruit? It's impossible to improve on Pogo's advice when he said, "We've identified the enemy and the enemy is us." Most people cause their own atheromatous plaques by faulty lifestyle, which starts at an early age.

The first move is to throw away cigarettes. Carbon monoxide in cigarette smoke causes blood platelets to adhere to the endothelial lining of arteries. This produces local injury and eventually atherosclerosis. Smoking also decreases the amount of oxygen in the blood, has an abnormal effect on the blood's fatty acids, and causes arterial spasm.

Have a regular medical checkup to make certain the blood pressure is normal. Too much pressure damages the inside of a hose. It does the same thing to arteries, and when damage occurs, atherosclerosis is not far behind.

Keep your weight under control. Obesity is a cause of diabetes, which in turn accelerates the development of atherosclerosis. A high-fiber diet, limited calories, and regular exercise will all help to keep arteries open.

One final word for young readers. Don't wait until you're 60 to climb the stairs instead of taking an elevator, and toss the sugar bowl and salt shaker off the table. Atherosclerosis is never forgiving of past sins. A careful, balanced lifestyle must be a lifelong habit.

The Earlobe Crease: A Prime Indicator of Heart Disease

Is it possible to diagnose coronary heart disease (CHD) without the aid of electrocardiograms and other twentieth-century technology? To predict atherosclerosis of the coronary vessels by an examination that takes just one second, is painless, and has an accuracy of about 75 percent? Sounds incredible. But the earlobe crease is proclaimed by some physicians to be the window to the heart.

Dr. William Elliot at Washington University School of Medicine has examined 1,000 patients with coronary heart disease. His studies reveal that 74 percent of the patients with CHD have this peculiar earlobe crease. Only 16 percent without the crease suffered from CHD.

The Washington University study is not an isolated one. Similar studies covering 6,500 patients showed that 60 percent of those with the earlobe crease had heart disease.

Dr. Elliot says the crease starts where the earlobe attaches to the head and angles diagonally towards the back edge of the ear. Some patients have a faint crease. Others a deep and obvious one. It can be present in one or both ears.

What causes the earlobe crease? The earlobe is one of the thinnest and softest parts of the body. It's also well supplied with small blood vessels called arterioles. Researchers in Poland, Finland, and Israel say degeneration of the elastic material around the earlobe arterioles causes the crease. This is the same type of change that's associated with hardening of the arteries in the heart.

Not all doctors agree with Dr. Elliot. His critics contend the arterial disease-crease relationship is purely coincidental. They point out that many of the patients were in hospital being treated for CHD anyway. Others claim the earlobe crease is simply more common in older people, who are more likely to have blocked coronary vessels.

Are these arguments valid ones? Dr. Elliot says studies have also been done on hospital patients being treated for conditions unrelated to the heart, and age has been taken into consideration. But there continues to be a strong association between the earlobe crease and CHD.

Dr. Elliot has another ace card up his sleeve. Autopsies on young accident victims show that CHD due to atherosclerosis often begins at an early age in North America. But it rarely makes its presence felt until later on in life. The earlobe crease is similarly an acquired abnormality rarely seen in young people. So far this sign has been reported in just two people under the age of 30; both of them had CHD. In another study all but four patients under 40 with the earlobe crease were found to have CHD.

Dr. Elliot calls his findings significant, but not earth-shattering. He says it won't make any difference in the way doctors practice medicine. But he believes the sign is a valid one and that physicians should look for it. After all, it's one of the few things today that doesn't cost anything and it takes just a second or two to spot.

I had some hesitation about writing this column. It brought visions of readers rushing to the mirror to see if an earlobe crease was present, then worrying themselves to death if they found one.

But I don't believe in hiding facts, and Dr. Elliot has made an astute observation. As well, the accuracy of the earlobe crease in predicting CHD impresses me, particularly at a time when everyone worships machines. The routine measurement of a patient's cholesterol level and blood pressure, assessments of his weight, smoking habits, and personality type have worse records of predictability than the simple earlobe crease.

So you can't resist a look? Remember the earlobe crease is still just a clue that provides a tip-off for possible CHD but isn't a definite diagnosis. Discovering an earlobe crease could also be a blessing in disguise for some patients. Especially those who are going to start a better lifestyle next week. Or the week following.

6

Cancer

Some letters from readers make my blood boil every year. Not the kind asking if it's worth $25 an hour to sit in a uranium mine to cure rheumatism; I agree with P.T. Barnum there's a sucker born every minute, and it's impossible to be your brother's keeper. The ones I hate are those from parents whose children have cancer. Or from adults with a fatal malignancy. These letters always ask what I think of a particular cancer remedy—never remedies suggested by recognized medical doctors, but from someone who claims to be a doctor of "metaphysics" or some other fictitious title. These charlatans should be strung up by their thumbs. Preying on the desperate is a despicable way to make a living. And the public shouldn't have to fall prey to them.

The most tragic incident on record involves Linda Epping, an eight-year-old child with a cancerous growth in one eye. Doctors believed they could save the child's life by speedy removal of the eye. But her parents met a woman in the waiting room of the California Medical Center in Los Angeles.

The woman told the Eppings that her son's tumor had been cured without surgery by a chiropractor. Linda's parents, distraught at this point, removed the child from hospital and placed her under the care of Marvin Phillips, the chiropractor. She received vitamins, large amounts of unidentified pills, enemas, and special exercises. But the cancer continued to grow. Desperate again, the parents eventually returned her to the hospital, where she soon died. Phillips was convicted of second-degree murder and sent to jail.

But one or a dozen convictions don't stop charlatanism. Year after year it's estimated that over two billion dollars go down the drain for worthless cancer cures. Economic loss is one thing. But false hopes and delays in early diagnosis cause immeasurable damage.

The *Cancer Journal for Clinicians* reveals a range of ludicrous treatments that are foisted on the public every day. The simpler ones involve corrosive or caustic agents used to treat external cancer. One remedy recommended natural products such as cobwebs saturated with arsenic to be applied as a poultice. This would supposedly draw out any malignancy.

Other quacks claim that cancer is caused by impurities. They advise a strict diet to detoxify and rid the body of these substances. To accomplish this they advocate a raw food diet. A diet of grapes is supposed to work a marvelous cure.

Beware if the "doctor's" office looks more like a TV repair shop than a medical office. It's unbelievable the extent to which some people can be fooled. One quack in Los Angeles stated he could diagnose all disease from a drop of a patient's blood. He claimed blood crystals would activate his machine to a certain wave length. This astounding machine would then broadcast "healing waves" to patients hundreds of miles away.

Cancer quackery isn't a new problem. In 1794 General George Washington publicly commended a Mrs. Johnson for her recipe to cure cancer. The remedy? A mixture of garden sorrel, celandine, persimmon bark, and spring water.

The discovery of electricity started the golden age of quackery. In 1795 Dr. Elisha Perkins introduced his "metallic tractors," made from different kinds of metal. The two metals would remove poisonous electrical fluid, which was the basis of all suffering. The tractors were merely passed over affected parts of the body to yank out disease. The gullible George Washington was one of Dr. Perkins's patients.

Since that time hundreds of other worthless products have been promoted as cures for cancer—substances prepared from pooled cancer tissue of animals, or products prepared from a patient's own blood and urine.

Remember that charlatans are usually very personable, friendly individuals. That's all they have to sell. But they're wolves in sheep's clothing. They are well aware of the desperation of cancer patients and their families. They know that such people will clutch at straws. The quack makes a living by exploiting this fear.

For many, quackery offers an escape from reality. We all like to believe that wishes come true. The threat of one's own death or the death of a loved one can drive the intelligent into a world of make-believe. A desperate search for a therapeutic miracle can twist facts to suit emotional needs. This may soothe the psyche temporarily, but it does not cure cancer. The only salvation remains the same. If cancer is suspected, get a reputable medical diagnosis quickly and follow the treatment prescribed by a licensed physician. If cure does not then follow, fairy tales will not help either.

Can You Inherit Cancer?

"My father died from cancer of the lung several years ago. Now my mother has passed away from breast cancer. Does this mean I'm going to get cancer?" Every year I receive letters asking me this question. Can cancer be inherited? What does it really mean when cancer strikes family members?

Doctors usually say cancer isn't inherited. This is meant to reassure patients that there's no need to worry about being unusually susceptible to this dreaded disease. It's generally a correct statement. But facts now show that some families are at greater risk. And it's a disservice not to tell them. Forewarned is forearmed.

We know that retinoblastomas of the eye and Wilm's tumors of the kidney have been traced to chromosomal defects. Cancer of the stomach is seen more frequently in people with group A blood. And children with Down's syndrome have a higher rate of leukemia. But what about the better-known malignancies?

Lung cancer, the most common malignancy in males, will soon be the major one in females. Today most people associate this disease with smoking. But it appears genetics also plays a role here. One study revealed that non-smokers with a family history of lung cancer were four times more likely to develop this malignancy than non-smokers with no family history of the problem. Moreover smokers with a family history of lung cancer had 14 times more risk of this disease than smokers with no family history of the malignancy.

Cancer of the large bowel (colon) is the second most common malignancy in this country. One type associated with polyps (stalklike projections of the bowel tissue into the center of the intestine) is inherited as a dominant disease. It means that if a parent has this disease, the children have a 50 percent chance of being affected. But luckily the great majority of large bowel cancers are not inherited.

How does genetics affect breast cancer? We know that family members are at greater risk if their mother or sister had cancer of the breast. But recent research shows that the danger is also related to the age at which relatives were affected and whether the malignancy occurred in one or both breasts.

For instance, if the malignancy occurred in both breasts and started before the menopause, sisters or daughters of such patients have a nine times greater chance of getting this disease. But if both your mother and sister had breast cancer in each breast at an early age, the risk jumps to about 40 times the normal rate.

There are also well-documented cases of what has been labeled "the family cancer syndrome." Such families have cancers of various types, predominantly malignancies of the breast, uterus, ovary, and large bowel. They are also noted for having multiple malignancies. These cancers occur at unusually early ages.

Never forget that cancer causes about 25 per cent of the deaths in North America. Consequently it's not surprising that by chance alone malignancy can strike several members of a family. The majority of cancers are therefore not inherited. Rather, they result from the interaction of genes and the environment. This is where smart consumers can decrease their chances of succumbing to malignancy.

In 1849 in London, England, John Snow turned off the Broad Street pump valve, preventing sewage-contaminated water from infecting parts of the city with cholera. You can't turn off all the valves causing cancer quite so easily. But how much more evidence do consumers need before they slam shut the valve that sends cancerous smoke into their lungs?

Families with a history of colon cancer should increase their dietary intake of vitamin C, calcium, and fiber. They should quickly report rectal bleeding, black stools, or a change in bowel habits to their doctor. Stools should be tested for microscopic blood at regular intervals. And the bowel should be examined by the flexible colonoscope (lighted instrument) once a year.

Women with a family history of breast cancer should routinely perform self-examination of the breasts every month. They should quickly report any lump, swelling, change in the shape of the breast, discharge from the nipple, or retraction of the nipple to the doctor. A baseline mammogram (x-ray) of the breasts should be done between the ages of 35 and 40. And over 40 years of age regular mammograms are needed to detect early cancer changes in the breast.

Breast Cancer—The Cause and the Diagnosis

Breast cancer is still one of the world's greatest unconquered killers. The figures show the immensity of the problem. In Canada and the United States there are 25 million females over 25 years of age; four million of these women will eventually develop a breast malignancy. It means that every year there are 90,000 new cases and that half of these patients will be dead within 10 years. And despite modern technology, 95 percent of patients still find the cancer with their own fingers. What causes this malignancy and can some cases be prevented?

There is a tremendous amount of conflicting evidence as to what may trigger this disease. For example, some experts believe that it makes no difference whether or not women breastfeed their infants.

Other doctors disagree. They report that in China, India, and Japan mothers who by tradition nurse children have fewer cancers of the breast. This relationship has also been noted in Israel. The Jews of Asian origin customarily nurse their babies and have less breast cancer than Jews of European origin, who often reject breast feeding.

French Canadians have also added some weight to this theory. In 1970 the death rate from breast cancer in Quebec was the greatest in the world. At that time only 18 percent of mothers nursed their children. But there is one other factor to consider in Quebec. Some experts reflect that the large number of Catholic nuns might be partly responsible for this high figure. Several studies have shown that women who never become pregnant are more prone to breast cancers. Similarly women who postpone having a child until the mid-30s are also higher-risk candidates for this disease.

Many women ask if breast cancer can be inherited. No one has ever proven that the genes for this disease can be passed from one generation to the other. But there is a rather disquieting tendency for breast cancer to run in certain families. For example, the average woman has 1 chance in 15 of developing the problem. But if a grandmother, mother, or sister had the disease, the probability changes to about one in seven. And if both mother and sister had breast cancer the chance is even greater.

No doctor would disagree that age is also a predisposing factor. Like the majority of malignancies, breast cancer is reasonably rare in the young. The greatest number of cases occur between 40 and 60 years of age. Moreover, some studies have shown that women in their 70s who discover a breast lump have an 80 percent chance of it being a cancer. Earlier in life the probability is only about 20 percent.

Diet has been implicated as a causative factor. Breast cancer is more common in countries like Canada and the U.S., where people consume large amounts of animal fat, and where obesity is fast becoming the number one disease. Is that the reason why Japanese women who move to North America and change their dietary habits develop more breast cancer than those who stay at home?

Does a virus cause breast cancer? Animal experiments show that a virus can be transmitted in mother's milk, producing this disease. If the mice are removed from their mothers at birth, they do not get this malignancy.

There is no definite evidence that this happens in humans. But virus particles similar to those that cause cancer in mice have been found in the milk of the Parsis of Bombay. These women have four times as many breast cancers as other women of this city. It's therefore been suggested by some doctors that women with a strong family history of breast cancer should not nurse babies.

Could it be that sometimes nursing helps to prevent breast cancer, but triggers it in other women? At the moment no one knows the answer. Speculating on these theories is interesting. But it's more practical for patients to diagnose breast cancer at the earliest time. Right now, that is the only sure way to achieve a 100 percent cure.

Remember that early breast cancer doesn't cause pain. You must therefore develop the habit of using your own fingers to find small lumps. Get to know what your breast feels like at different times of the month. If you notice a change, never, never wait and hope it will go away. This is the reason why so many thousands of women die from the disease. And if you have a doctor who never examines your breasts, find another one who will do it.

Mammography

What will future historians say about today's mammography—breast x-rays to detect small breast cancers (SBCs)? Will they conclude it's been a dangerous tool which triggers more cancer than it cures? That routine breast examination is still the best way to diagnose breast cancer? Or that mammography can and does save lives from this dread disease?

Breast malignancy is still the number one killer of middle-aged women. One in every 11 women born today will eventually develop cancer of the breast; one in five of these will die from it. It's a chilling fact that during the last 30 years advances in surgery haven't significantly reduced the death rate from cancer of the breast.

The conclusion is obvious. The only successful way to fight this disease is by early diagnosis. This means detecting small breast cancers before they can be felt by patients or doctors.

Dr. David D. Paulus, a professor at the University of Texas, is an expert on mammography. He claims that it is the only reliable means of spotting SBCs. And that 95 percent of patients with minimal breast cancers diagnosed by this method will be alive in 10 years.

But how often does mammography pick up SBCs that are not felt by physicians? The National Cancer Institute and the American Cancer Society recently screened 261,859 women who had no symptoms of the disease. Mammography discovered 734 breast cancers. Researchers concluded that half of these malignancies would have been missed by doctors. And 40 percent of the patients were under 50 years of age.

When, then, is the right age to consider having a mammogram? Dr. Allan Bassett, director of the breast screening clinic at Mount Sinai Hospital, Toronto, never performs mammography on women under 35 years of age. Breast tissue, he says, is simply too dense and obscures any SBCs that may be present. This same dense breast tissue also sometimes gives the false impression that a cancer is present. This results in too many needless biopsies of the breast and, in turn, frightens women unnecessarily when cancer is not present. Mammography should therefore be reserved for women over 40 years of age. It's also the age when the majority of breast cancers begin to occur. How frequently mammograms are taken depends on whether the patient is in a low- or high-risk category.

Women who have never had a child have a slightly higher risk of breast malignancy. This also holds for women who start a family late in life or have prolonged menstrual activity. A woman who has menstruated for 40 years or more has twice the risk as one who has menstruated for only 30 years. Obesity also tends to favor the occurrence of this disease.

Females with fibrocystic disease of the breast also have a considerably higher risk. So have patients with a family history of breast cancer, particularly if it involved a mother or sister. But this familial relationship does not always hold true. In addition, patients who have a malignancy removed from one breast have a 15 times greater chance it will occur in the other breast. And if a mammogram detects an abnormal architectural pattern in the breast, such as fine clusters of calcification, it immediately places the patient in a very high-risk category.

Patients and doctors must remember that mammography cannot substitute for regular breast examinations. No test is perfect, and mammography sometimes misses lesions that can be felt. Moreover, if a lump is palpable it must be treated immediately, regardless of mammogram findings. Treatment may involve only simple needle aspiration of the breast rather than surgical removal.

How do I treat my patients? I ask them to fill out a questionnaire to determine their risk of breast cancer. At 40 years of age I recommend an initial routine mammogram. The frequency of future mammograms depends on the condition of the breasts and the risk factor of the patient. But after 50 years of age annual mammograms are prescribed.

Today's improved techniques assure that the amount of radiation received (¼ rad) during this treatment is 40 times less than the radiation given in former years. It's estimated that a level of one rad might induce one case of malignancy in one million women. But the failure to do mammography denies early diagnosis to 1,350 patients. Thus the value of mammography far outweighs its risk.

Doctors who use mammography, however, have a major responsibility. They should refer their patients only to centers where the equipment is monitored regularly by physicists to detect excessive radiation exposure. If we follow this approach I believe future historians will treat us kindly. It is, after all, the only tool we have to diagnose SBCs.

What Moles Should Be Removed to Prevent Cancer?

"How can you be so cheap?" a surgical colleague asked me. He caught me in the act of removing my own mole from my side in the hospital's emergency department. It wasn't because I wanted to avoid his fee. I just decided on the spur of the moment to excise a bothersome mole, one that was being constantly irritated by my belt. His question made me think about this common problem: How can you distinguish between unimportant and dangerous moles, and why do people still die from a cancer that is so easily prevented?

I'm not suggesting a stampede across the country to remove every mole. Most people have between 15 and 20 of these benign skin lesions. But there's been an increase in the number of cancerous moles in the 20- to 40-year age group. And more people are dying from this disease than in former years.

No race, sex, or age group is immune to malignant moles, but some people have to be particularly careful. For instance, Australians have the highest reported incidence of malignant moles in the world. Indians are more prone to get them on the soles of their feet. Blacks have five times as many as whites. And sandy-haired persons who freckle easily are more susceptible to this form of cancer.

How can you spot a dangerous mole? It's not always easy, because, like the automobile, there is a variety of types. They may be flat, slightly raised, or have a small pedicule. The mole may or may not contain hair. They also come in a multitude of colors. Some are the normal shade of the skin. Others are coal black or darker around the outside of the mole. Still others contain a mixture of white, purple, blue, and red. Nearly all have indefinite margins and often there's a red inflammation around the periphery of the mole. In some cases small satellite moles exist in the immediate vicinity.

Pigmented moles appear early in life. In males they reach a peak at about age 30. Females have the highest number by 40. During adolescence it's rare for a mole to cause trouble.

Some malignant moles occur in normal skin, but two-thirds originate from an existing mole. Initially the mole increases locally in size. But it eventually spreads to lymph nodes and distant organs such as the liver and lungs. In half the cases the heart becomes involved.

How can you prevent a mole from becoming cancerous? The only way is to remove suspicious ones and those in high-risk locations. For instance, constant trauma may trigger a malignant change. That's why it's sound preventive medicine to excise moles which are constantly rubbed by a bra strap, belt, or shoe.

Don't hesitate to see your doctor if a mole starts to increase in size or changes color. There's a common misconception that questionable moles always get darker, but a malignancy can also be heralded when a mole takes on a lighter hue.

There are other signs that should flash on the red light. Most cancerous moles are without symptoms in the early stages. But sometimes a malignant change causes itching and a tingling sensation. You should also be very suspicious of smooth moles that become rough and scaly, or when one becomes tender, ulcerated, and bleeds easily.

Few people should die from a malignant mole. You don't require fancy equipment to look at the skin. Moreover, moles don't change overnight, so there's ample time to excise the lesion. Yet people continue to die from this disease because of a variety of errors.

Procrastination by doctors and patients kills many people. Don't say, "I'll have it removed one of these days." That normally means it will never be done. Or when it is finally cut out the cancer will have already spread to other organs.

To find a questionable mole you also have to look for it. But the family doctor may be too busy practicing assembly-line medicine to spot the lesion. The internist may be too occupied reading the electrocardiogram. And the gynecologist may be too engrossed with the pelvic examination. While all this is going on, the lethal culprit may be lurking beneath a bra strap.

Sometimes the reverse is true. The mole has been staring a variety of doctors in the eye for years, but each one leaves it for someone else to remove.

Make moles your own business. Make sure the doctor examines large or questionable moles during an office visit. And if there's ever any doubt about the mole, the best move is to have it cut out. To everyone's surprise some moles that are removed for purely cosmetic reasons are reported malignant by the pathologist.

Unfortunately medicine is at times like politics and economics. Everyone knows how to cure the problem. But who does anything about it?

Handling the Psychological Impact of Cancer

How do most people react when the doctor tells them they've got cancer? During 1982, 900,000 North Americans received this diagnosis. Families and friends should be aware of the various ways patients respond to this shocking news.

Hearing a physician say, "We've found a malignancy," poses a unique and special threat. Usually a predictable series of disorganized thoughts flies through the mind. How will family and friends react? Will we be treated differently and possibly isolated? Will there be loss of esteem? Will it affect our body image, sex lives, and lifestyle? Will we die? And how soon?

How one reacts to cancer depends partly on which organ is involved. The Memorial Hospital for Cancer and Allied Diseases studied this problem. Dr. Arthur M. Sutherland reports in the *Cancer Journal for Clinicians* that colostomy patients often fear the disapproval of society, as they once worried about criticism from a toilet-training mother. One patient was described by her family as a "crazy-clean housekeeper." She developed cancer of the rectum and reluctantly agreed to surgery. But when she discovered that a colostomy was required, she became depressed and contemplated suicide. She believed she was unacceptable to friends and eventually isolated herself. To her, life became worthless.

Predicting how a patient will react is an uncertain task. Many of us would be hard pressed to know what goes on in the mind of a best friend under normal circumstances. It's therefore difficult for surgeons to forecast how people will compensate for the loss of a breast, leg, or bowel function. There's a wide range of possibilities.

The initial response is often a refusal to accept the diagnosis. Fear of cancer is so intense that it must be removed from consciousness. The patient rationalizes that the doctor is wrong. Conversely, the threat to existence may be so overwhelming that some patients want to rush headlong into surgery. Others find a dozen illogical reasons to postpone an operation. They ask, "Why multilate my body if I'm going to die in a few months anyway?"

After surgery, patients may fall into one of several pitfalls. One man was convinced the cancer of the prostate gland he had developed was a form of punishment. During his life he had enjoyed several extramarital affairs; now he felt he was reaping the reward of immoral behavior.

The Memorial Hospital study cites another problem. Hypochondriacs, those who fear disease, usually approach surgery expecting the worst to happen. Post-operatively many believe that irreparable damage has been done. They are convinced that removal of any part of their body decreases vital energy, thus rendering them more susceptible to the recurrence of malignancy. As a result, they rigidly restrict all activity, believing they are thus prolonging their lives. It is a pattern that is difficult for physicians to break. As one patient remarked, "I treat my body like an old car. I expect it to break down any minute."

Some hypochondriacs develop paranoid reactions. They're convinced the surgeon made an error. Or that the operation was more extensive than it needed to be. Such thoughts can lead to a descent into depression and, on rare occasions, suicide.

Obsessive-compulsive reactions are usually seen in patients who have rectal surgery resulting in colostomy. All patients who undergo colostomy develop this to some degree. But those who were compulsive about body habits prior to surgery may experience exaggerated reactions. One man was compelled to spend hours every day irrigating the colostomy. He needed to be sure it was clean before seeing friends.

Families should realize that some cancer patients are very demanding. They often complain of minor symptoms and aggravations. This is an attempt to distract themselves from the anxiety of cancer and possible death.

It's been said that fear is the greatest of all inventors. A minor post-operative complication may be perceived by the patient as a recurrence of malignancy. A few words of explanation by doctors and nurses can prevent hours or days of anguish. Similarly, experienced enterostomal therapists can now ease the apprehension of colostomy. But most of all, honest and supportive families or friends can help the patient make a gradual adjustment to the diagnosis of cancer.

Lifestyle and Cancer Prevention

Pogo was right; "The enemy is us." Every year 500,000 North Americans succumb to cancer. We know now that 60 to 80 percent of these malignancies can be prevented by a change in lifestyle. The sobering thought is that doctors might discover the cause of every type of cancer, yet still be unable to prevent a single case. Most people still refuse to adopt an anti-cancer lifestyle. But is this careless lifestyle to which so many of us cling really worth dying for?

Cancer, like obesity, is a disease of civilization. People generally believe that being overweight may increase the risk of heart attack and that's all. But the American Cancer Society reports that when people are 40 percent above their ideal weight, the incidence of cancer rises dramatically. It's 55 percent higher than normal for obese women, showing increased rates of breast, uterine, and ovarian malignancies. For overweight men there is a 33 percent increase in cancer.

Several possible reasons for this association emerge. Obese people eat more and therefore consume greater quantities of food additives that have a carcinogenetic effect. They also tend to consume a high-fat, high-red-meat diet, which has also been implicated in cancer.

Obese women manufacture excess quantities of estrogen in their fatty tissues. Some researchers believe that this constant barrage of estrogen year after year is a factor in breast and uterine cancer.

A change in sexual habits might also reduce certain types of malignancy. Tentative findings indicate that women who are exposed sexually to herpes simplex II virus are more likely to develop cancer of the cervix (the opening into the uterus).

Homosexuals are at greater risk. Those who have a lifestyle involving many sexual partners have a high incidence of skin cancer called Kaposi's sarcoma, as well as rectal cancer and Burkitt's lymphoma. Common sense demands that it pays to ask a sexual partner whether he or she has ever suffered from herpes, to restrict the number of sexual partners, and to remember that condoms may still be the best means of protection from herpes infection.

Women who remarry face another risk. Male semen carries the potential for triggering cancer of the cervix. If, for instance, a first wife died of this disease, the second wife has three to four times the chance of developing the same malignancy. The best precaution in this case is an annual Pap smear.

How many martinis before dinner may we consume before increasing the risk of malignancy? It's been aptly said that, "One swallow does not make a summer, but too many swallows a fall." Studies show that cancer of the windpipe is 10 times higher in those who drink, cancer of the foodpipe 25 times more common in heavy drinkers. They key word is moderation. And if you do drink, don't waste the alcohol quota on mouthwashes. Two separate reports indicate that habitual users of strongly alcoholic mouthwashes face higher rates of oral cancer.

Never forget this fact. Cancer of the lung, breast, and large bowel account for 46 percent of all malignancies. Dietary changes and elimination of cigarette smoking would eradicate 50 percent of these cancers.

During World War II in England there was a shortage of sugar, dairy products, and meat. The English substituted cereals and vegetables. This simple action caused a sharp drop in breast cancer. But after the war when citizens returned to earlier dietary habits, the rate of breast cancer returned to former levels.

Fiber is an impressive way to fight malignancy of the large bowel. Fiber holds water and greases the intestines, thereby decreasing the transit time of food through the bowel. This gets rid of our own garbage quicker, leaving less time for cancer-causing substances to act on the bowel wall.

Vitamins A, C, and E should be consumed in adequate amounts. People who eat vitamin A foods regularly have less lung and other cancers. Vitamin E also helps to hinder the production of carcinogenic nitrosamines in the stomach and intestines. Zinc in cereals and selenium in seafoods may also be protective against malignancy.

Most people tend to say, "Why bother changing your lifestyle? If it isn't coffee that causes cancer, it's the nitrates in hot dogs. Or the nitrosamines in beer. So the hell with it."

I agree that it's foolish to try to live in a glass cage. But surely it makes sense to try a healthier diet, to drink in moderation, and to toss away cigarettes, the most virulent of cancer causing products. Even Pogo would champion such obvious changes in lifestyle.

Motherhood Rules Help Fight Cancer

What is the best way to diagnose cancer? Should a patient rely totally on the expertise of a family doctor? Are there occasions when he or she should think "This treatment doesn't make sense. Maybe my doctor has had a tough day and is tired. Am I being misled by a physician who should know better? Would it be wise to obtain another opinion?" How you answer these questions could save your life.

Doctors sometimes display a glaring lack of horse sense. For example, a male tennis partner recently said to me, "I went to see my doctor because of a breast lump. He said that cancer of the breast is rare in males, and I should return in three months. But the lump is still present. What do you think I should do?"

This man hadn't played a single game of tennis since finding the lump. Instead he'd spent the summer contemplating his possible demise. Why? Because his physician had forgotten that certain facts about cancer, like motherhood, are sacred.

Dr. David Klaassen is associated with the Cancer Foundation. He made this point during an interview with Peter De Vries of the *Medical Post*: "We find it's the basic principles which are broken time and time again when the problems occur."

For example, it's an accepted dictum that breast lumps should receive immediate attention. Some physicians prefer to aspirate cystic breast lumps in women. Others believe that all lumps should be excised. Few would decide to leave a breast lump unattended in either sex.

One observation of Dr. Klaassen's made me smile. He commented, "Most internists think the breasts are something you throw out of the way when you listen to the heart." But it takes only a few seconds to examine a breast. And patients often tell me that neither family doctor nor specialist has bothered to check their breasts for lumps. Everyone assumes that someone else is going to do it. Specialists can be so engrossed in their own field of medicine they can't see the forest for the trees.

"Motherhood" axioms about cancer have assumed a new dimension in the 1980s. Life has become more complex for both the doctor and the patient. Physicians have a variety of new diagnostic tests at their disposal. But if doctors don't use the proven common sense approach, lethal errors can be made.

For instance, mammography is being used more and more to diagnose early breast malignancies. But cancer clinics are encountering a new problem. A patient may consult a doctor because of a breast lump and then undergo mammography. The mammogram may be reported as normal and so nothing further is done. Later it's discovered the patient has advanced cancer because the doctor relied totally on a new test. He should have exercised common sense and removed the lump.

Blind faith in a new technique is one pitfall for both doctors and patients. Failing to use a well-established diagnostic routine is another. Patient X consulted his doctor because of rectal bleeding. The cause of the bleeding seemed obvious. Large hemorrhoids were present. The patient was told he'd eventually need a hemorrhoidectomy.

But his doctor had side-stepped another "motherhood" principle. He failed to order a barium enema x-ray. Nor did he insert a lighted instrument to explore the large bowel and detect less obvious reasons for bleeding. Several months later this patient developed an acute bowel obstruction. An emergency operation revealed a large malignancy of the lower intestine that had spread to other organs.

To err is a human trait. But it's a big mistake when neglect of simple, routine procedures causes needless death. Abnormal bleeding at the time of "change of life" is usually due to hormonal upset. But it can also be the result of early malignancy. A physician who writes it off as due to menopause without a D and C (scraping the inside of the uterus) is ignoring another motherhood principle.

No one should play Russian roulette with potentially dangerous symptoms. Difficulty swallowing, hoarseness, a persistent cough all demand a thorough investigation. So does the passage of bloody urine, an ulcer that fails to heal, or a mole that changes in size and colour.

It's been said that hasty climbers have sudden falls. Shortcuts in cancer diagnosis can be equally hazardous. Patients, like my tennis friend, deserve a second opinion. If an error or omission is made, no matter how inadvertent, it's the patient who suffers. There's much truth in the Hindu saying, "Whether the knife falls on the melon or the melon on the knife, the melon suffers."

A Hell of a Way to Achieve Equality

For years women have fought justifiably for equal rights. Now statistics show that by 1990 they will have achieved it in one area at least. But it's a hell of a way to be equal. Like males, they'll share lung cancer as their number one killer. Breast malignancies will drop to second spot. Women, it seems, have been caught by the old adage "Give someone enough rope and she'll hang herself."

A graph published in the February 1981 *Cancer Journal for Clinicians* dramatically illustrated the problem. There's been a sharp decrease in the number of female deaths from cancer of the uterus and stomach, but for the past 15 years a steady increase in the number of women dying from cancer of the lung.

The atomic bomb, dropped on Hiroshima and Nagasaki, revealed an important fact about cancer. Two irritants are worse than one. The bomb's radiation initiated lung cancer. But the citizens of these stricken cities who also smoked developed more malignancies of the lung.

North American women are now subject to a similar double whammy. More are smoking as well as being exposed to industrial carcinogens. It's a lethal combination.

Pulmonary irritants, like asbestos, have been injuring men's lungs for years. Today females are inhaling an equal number of cancer-related pollutants. For example, 35,000 women working in the meat-packing industry are exposed to dangerous gases in meat wrappings. The plastic film used to seal meat is melted by a hot wire. This produces hydrochloric acid and phosgene fumes, causing a recurrent respiratory illness called "meat packer's asthma." Another 500,000 women are working in the plastics and rubber industry. They're exposed to talc dust and carbon black, both pulmonary irritants.

Dozens of other situations could be cited. Vinyl chloride is one of the most widely used chemicals in the U.S. It's known to cause liver cancer. It's also suspicious in the occurrence of lung malignancies. Until recently it was used as a propellant in household and cosmetic products, usually to be sprayed in poorly ventilated bathrooms and laundry areas.

How much of this double exposure affects lung cancer is unknown at the moment. But common sense dictates that smothering lung tissue with multiple carcinogens is a risky game. And the earlier it begins the greater the potential for lung cancer.

Teenagers who start smoking discount recklessly the inherent dangers of this habit. It's frustrating to see them puffing themselves into eventual agony. We send rockets to Mars. We've developed a technology beyond the wildest dreams of our forefathers. But we are helpless in communicating the horrendous facts of smoking to teenagers of both sexes.

Recently I watched one of my patients die painfully of lung cancer. It's always a terrible sight and I was depressed. On the way home I spotted a group of young girls smoking on the steps of their high school. I had an overwhelming desire to take them back to the hospital and show them first hand what might happen to them in the future. But I knew it was a hopeless task.

These girls and most adults have no conception of what it means to develop lung cancer. Dr. Eugene P. Fazzini of the New York University School of Medicine puts it as well as anyone. He writes, "The natural history of lung cancer is that of a rapidly fatal tumor with few patients surviving as long as two years from the time of the diagnosis. The overall five-year survival rate is 5 to 7 percent." That says it all.

Why is the outcome so disastrous? There's one obvious reason. Early cancer of the lung has no symptoms. Malignancy is always well established by the time patients begin to complain of a persistent cough, increased amounts of sputum, blood in the sputum, or chest pain.

Dr. G. H. Bayle was the first doctor to describe lung cancer in the nineteenth century. But it wasn't until 1933 that Drs. E. A. Graham and J. Singer removed a cancerous lung. We haven't made much progress since then. Fifty to 75 percent of lung cancers have already spread by the time patients are seen by a doctor.

Predicting the outcome for the 80s is easy. Researchers are unlikely to develop a practical way to detect early lung cancer. The majority of people will continue to smoke. And the diagnosis of lung cancer will remain a death sentence for over 90 percent of its victims.

So let's plan a celebration to commemorate human stupidity, when lung malignancy becomes the number one killer of women. We need to record for history the day women achieved equality, joining men to become the architects of their own misfortune.

Incurable Cancer: The Horse May Learn to Fly

Is there any hope for people with incurable cancer? Patients suffering from widespread disease that's beyond the scope of surgery, radiation, and chemotherapy? Regrettably these people normally die. But some patients confound physicians by spontaneous remission. They prove that the king's horse can sometimes learn to fly.

Dr. F.W. Stewart in 1952 reported a fascinating case in the *Texas Journal of Reproductive Biology and Medicine*. Tests proved without question that a woman had an inoperable myosarcoma of the uterus. But in a matter of hours a sudden change occurred. She developed a high fever, rash, and an eosinophilia of the white blood corpuscles, all signs of an allergic reaction. The extensive tumor and cancerous fluid in the abdomen disappeared within a few days. Ten years later she was still alive and well.

Dr. D.W. Penner in 1953 told about a two-year-old boy with a cancer of the thigh. X-rays showed that the malignancy had destroyed part of the bony femur. The child's parents refused treatment. But five years later he was in perfect health without any evidence of malignant growth.

Spontaneous remissions also occur after incomplete treatment. Dr. William Boyd, Canada's late distinguished pathologist, documented the case of a nine-month-old child with a huge adrenal tumor. Part of the cancer was removed at the Hospital For Sick Children in Toronto. The remainder was left in the abdomen. But at 24 years of age the patient was as active as her twin sister. There are also numerous instances where removal of the primary cancer resulted in disappearance of distant metastases.

Professor Boyd mentions another example where the patient won the battle. In 1932 a 32-year-old man had surgery for cancer of the large bowel. In 1946 a cancerous growth appeared in the neck. It and another one in 1952 were excised. Subsequently in 1956 the victim became overly tired and lost weight. Surgeons discovered the 1932 cancer had recurred in its original location. Doctors removed the growth as before and yet again in 1961 a cancer of the rectum. In 1967 the patient was alive and well after living with the threat of cancer for 35 years.

Spontaneous remission may add many years to life. In 1952 a 23-year-old Montreal woman had radical surgery for removal of a malignant melanoma of the foot and cancerous metastases in the groin. She married against medical advice and became pregnant. The liver enlarged and metastatic lesions appeared on the leg. Doctors considered her case hopeless. But after pregnancy the liver returned to normal. The distant growths disappeared after the third baby. Two more children were born. In 1961 the tumor began to grow and the patient died in a few months.

Are these cases rare and questionable? Not at all. Dr. T.C. Everson reported another 119 patients in the Annuals of the New York Academy of Science. Spontaneous remissions occurred in 14 patients with cancer of the kidney. Unexplained and unexpected cures saved patients with uterine, bladder, breast, bone, and numerous other malignancies.

How does it happen? The answer to this question may solve the cancer mystery. Researchers currently believe these patients develop an immunological reaction against cancer cells. After all, we know the body can build up an immunity against polio, measles, and other infections. To explore this possibility, some interesting experiments were performed.

First, convict volunteers from Ohio State Penitentiary were selected. The scientists injected them with tumor cells. They discovered these caused only an inflammatory reaction. The destruction of cancer cells became more rapid when a second implantation of cancer was made. But when these cells were injected into patients already suffering from cancer they continued to grow in 13 out of 15 patients. The new tumors had to be removed a few weeks later.

There's another interesting point. If cancer cells are destroyed by electro-coagulation, the products of these degenerating cells are slowly absorbed into the body. This appears to increase a person's immunity. For example, 400 patients with inoperable cancer of the rectum were treated by incomplete electrocoagulation of the malignancy. The five-year survival rate was an astonishing 75 per cent.

What has the king's horse to do with spontaneous remission? I sometimes tell cancer patients this story. A criminal was sentenced to death by the king. But he obtained a reprieve by assuring the king he could teach His Majesty's horse to fly within a year. When friends criticized him for such an absurd promise he answered," Within a year the king may die. Or I may die. Or the horse may die. And in a year, who knows? Maybe the horse will learn to fly."

How Families Can Help the Terminal Cancer Patient

During our lifetimes everyone has to learn to cope with dire news. Some people lose their life's savings on a poor investment. Others watch the ax fall on their chances for a promotion. Still others have to accept the inconveniences of a long-term illness. But what about the ultimate in bad news? How do most people react to the threat of personal extinction? Just as important, what must their families be aware of during those final days?

Since I wrote the column "Don't play games with the cancer patient," I've received a number of letters from readers. Mr. D.G. of Toronto said, "I agree that none of us are good actors and that we can't and shouldn't skirt around the truth with cancer patients. But once they know the facts how do you handle the problem as their condition deteriorates?"

Mrs. L.W. of Edmonton wrote, "Thank goodness you've helped to remove the conspiracy of silence surrounding cancer patients. But do you have any advice about caring for the terminal patient? Is there anything that you should do or steer away from when the end is near? Your last article stopped short of this point."

How does the average person prepare for the final curtain call? Just like actors no one accepts it with any enthusiasm, and nearly everyone hopes to have the curtain raised for another bow or two. Yet just as there are rules for living, so are there certain guidelines for the dying patient and his family.

First of all, remember that practically every cancer patient who faces death initially denies the concept of personal extinction. The patient may be an astute businessman who could scan a balance sheet in a few seconds and quickly conclude that bankruptcy was inevitable. But this same executive who looks in the mirror every morning will continue to talk as if his declining state will go on indefinitely. Like the charge of the Light Brigade, it is a delicate mixture of faith, hope, and bravery.

This denial phase gives the patient's psyche a chance to play for a little more time and ready itself for the final battle. For most people it is strictly a transitory period in the relentless march towards death, but for the rare person denying can last to the bitter end. Families should let their loved one use this denial technique as long as they want to do so.

Sooner or later, however, death becomes an obvious conclusion for most people. Yet even at this stage some patients will make a personal deal with themselves for just a little more time. Some may want to attend a child's wedding. Others will have a great desire to be present at a family reunion or to squeeze through the Christmas season. Miraculously some will win one last final battle before losing the war.

One of the finest men I've had the pleasure of knowing won his last Waterloo. He had been one of the founders and prime movers of a company and with much pride he had watched it grow over the years. During that time he had always spent a few days with his fellow directors at a northern lodge for an annual think session.

One year, however, he was suddenly struck by a mortal illness, and it was still many weeks prior to the scheduled trip. Day after day he continued to fight his crippling disease and finally it appeared that the end was approaching. Yet he got out of his bed and was driven many miles to the meeting. He spent his last hours with his old friends and immediately died on returning home.

This man's family knew how much this last endeavor meant to him, and they went to extreme lengths to help arrange it. It is the best way to play the game when the patient has set his sights on a particular goal. Here actions spoke louder than words. Moreover, once the end arrived this patient's family received some comfort from having made the trip a reality.

Finally there comes a time when patients can no longer deny, bargain, or smile. Many become totally demoralized and depressed after further surgery, chemotherapy, or radiation. This is a time when often momentous guilt surfaces as they think about leaving children or of financial burdens facing their family. If and when that moment comes, let them talk openly about these problems. Equally important, try to show them how some of these difficulties can be solved.

Experts on dying say that most patients enter a final "silent depression" during the terminal days. It represents a necessary preparation for death, and there is no point in trying to talk them out of it. Remember that patients who struggle against death to the last fall of the curtain never die in peace.

Actions should always take the place of words as death begins to descend. What patients fear most at this time is total abandonment by the doctor and their family, so your physical presence becomes of vital importance to them. A stroke of the hair, holding the hand, and the quiet company of someone in the room helps to ease the feeling of impending isolation. Follow the philosophy of the Good Samaritan and never, never walk away from a dying patient.

How much help can you expect from your doctor? Some physicians will give much solace to families, but don't be too surprised if other doctors move away from the terminal patient. One study revealed, shockingly, that physicians were more fearful of death than the lay person. Another one showed that doctor's visits to dying cancer patients decreased in number and the length of time.

Winding down the clock of life is always a trying time for patients and their families, and it is impossible to lay down strict rules that apply to all occasions. Possibly Francis Peabody, a former professor of theology at Harvard, gave the wisest advice when he counselled, "The secret of care of the patient is caring for the patient."

7

Alcohol

Are you expecting too much of your liver? Is there a lifestyle that will prevent a fatty liver? Or death from cirrhosis? You can get a few clues by keeping an eye on a baboon, a Harvard professor, and the Canadian dollar.

Cirrhosis is now listed among the 10 leading causes of death, and it's fast becoming a serious middle-aged disease. In the 30- to 50-year age group, it's the number four killer behind heart disease, strokes, and cancer.

Why is the liver taking such a beating? Because it's the body's main garbage disposal unit. Ninety percent of the alcohol consumed by the human body must be detoxified by this organ. In addition, we live in an increasingly hazardous world. Each year the liver must work overtime to handle more and more poisons. People are subjected to multiple anesthetics today. Others inhale chemicals such as carbon tetrachloride. And we all swallow copper and other poisons every day.

What does alcohol do to the liver? Experiments on baboons and human volunteers produced surprising results. The subjects developed fatty livers from drinking moderate amounts of alcohol for 7 to 14 days. Keeping the baboons on alcohol for longer periods resulted in alcoholic hepatitis. In North America cirrhosis, the final stage of liver disease, develops in about 10 percent of heavy drinkers.

How can you protect your liver? First, don't be a steady drinker. Business executives who consistently down three-martini lunches may be headed for trouble. So are lonely housewives who routinely drink away the morning blues. Too often today the hand that rocks the cradle is shaking from excessive alcohol. People who rest their livers are less likely to develop progressive liver disease.

A famous Harvard professor became renowned for heavy imbibing. Finally he died, and medical colleagues gathered anxiously around the autopsy table to observe his liver, expecting to find a small, hard, scarred, cirrhotic organ. But the professor had the last laugh. It was as healthy as a newborn baby's. He was an alcoholic, but no fool. Every night he went to the Harvard Club and consumed a large steak.

A high-protein diet helps to protect the liver. That's why cirrhosis is more prevalent in parts of the world where the main diet consists of carbohydrate. Don't have a cup of coffee for breakfast, martinis for lunch, and a plate of spaghetti for dinner.

The falling Canadian dollar can also help to prevent cirrhosis, according to British researchers. They analyzed three centuries of English drinking habits. The nineteenth century was the peak of England's status as a world power. The Empire was strong, but British livers were not as alcohol consumption soared. The Englishman's liver received a rest between 1900 and 1950, when the economy faltered. But for the last 25 years British livers are again getting too much work. I don't know how much Canadians drank 300 years ago. But they've consumed more beer, wine, and spirits each year since 1966. And every year there are more deaths from cirrhosis. Possibly our feeble dollar will help to arrest this trend.

How much alcohol can be safely consumed? Some figures are reassuring. For example, one textbook on liver disease states, "Continuous ingestion of two-thirds of a bottle of whiskey daily for 10 years is required to develop severe liver damage."

Other authorities are less optimistic. They stress that men shouldn't consume more than 7½ ounces a day. There's worse news for females. Their limit is 2½ ounces. Does this imply the experts are male chauvinists once again putting women in their place? Possibly not. It's been found in France that women are more susceptible to liver disease than men. There is also some evidence for a similar difference in England.

The majority of heavy drinkers don't get cirrhosis. No one knows why this is the case. Possibly genetic, environmental, and nutritional factors protect them. The liver also has great power of regeneration. Give this organ a holiday from drinking and a damaged liver will usually bounce back. But don't wait until cirrhosis occurs. At this point there's little reward for virtue.

Sensible drinking is the best way to prevent a damaged liver. But if you can't say no to a three-martini lunch, never forget the Harvard professor. Apples may prevent some medical problems, but steaks seem to be the best defence against cirrhosis.

Social Drinking: How Much Is Too Much?

How much risk is involved in having a martini or two with lunch? Or cocktails and wine with the evening meal? Where does the pleasure end and the risk of cirrhosis, hypertension, heart disease, and cancer begin? And if you prefer wine, should you divide your weight by 30 to obtain the magic quota that is safe?

Several studies have shown that moderate drinkers have fewer heart attacks than abstainers or heavy drinkers. Alcohol has a protective affect on the heart by increasing the amount of high-density lipoproteins, the good cholesterol that helps to protect against atherosclerosis. Non-drinkers have a 30 percent greater chance of having a coronary attack than moderate drinkers.

Heavy alcohol consumption is related to cancer of the mouth, pharynx, larynx, esophagus (foodpipe), large bowel, thyroid gland, and liver. These rates are also higher in women, with a positive association between alcohol and rectal cancer.

But there's considerable doubt that moderate social drinking causes malignancy. As Robin Room of Berkeley's Alcohol Research Group remarks, "The man who goes to a ball game drinks beer that may facilitate cancer or even contain carcinogens such as asbestos fibers. But he may also have a soft drink that has carcinogens or a hot dog that has cancer-producing nitrites."

Social drinking can affect the blood pressure. The first two drinks raise the pressure, but it decreases above this amount. Yet more than two drinks a day does increase blood pressure over a long term. So if you have a family history of hypertension, be extra cautious about alcohol consumption.

Experts don't agree on how much is too much. Doctors Pequegnot and Tuyn at France's National Institute for Health believe the risk of developing cirrhosis from consuming 20 grams of alcohol a day is extremely small. This is the equivalent of ¼ liter of 10 percent wine, a pint of 5 percent beer, or 2 ounces of straight whiskey. But they stress that if you drink more you're not necessarily destined to get cirrhosis of the liver.

Dr. Thomas Turner of Johns Hopkins University allows more for social drinkers. He says, "Chronic ill effects in man are rare below a daily intake of 80 grams." He provides a formula for safe drinking: To determine the number of ounces of 80 proof spirits you can safely consume, divide your weight by 30. A 150-pound man could therefore consume 5 ounces of liquor daily. For 12 percent wine, divide your weight by nine; for beer divide it by three.

Today the general trend in alcohol research tends to implicate smaller and smaller amounts of alcohol in health problems, however. For instance, researchers have shown that even a single dry martini substantially increases the fat in the liver which is visible under the microscope. Too much social drinking over the years can lead to a fatty liver, which may progress to cirrhosis.

What is the safe way to drink? Most authorities agree that two drinks a day of liquor, or a glass of wine, or two beers, is not too much and is probably good preventive medicine.

Wine and beer also seem to have the edge on hard liquor. The World Health Organization reports that deaths from cirrhosis are 50 percent greater with consumption of spirits than with wine or beer.

Remember that the more concentrated the alcohol the greater the irritant effects. So if you must have whiskey, dilute it. And stay away from martinis, manhattans, and drinks "on-the-rocks."

Weekend spree drinkers also have four times the mortality rate of those who spread out their drinking. So if you are determined to take 14 drinks a week, it's safer to take two every day.

Be sure to confine your drinking to one occasion a day. Men who drink both at lunch and again at dinner have a 70 percent higher mortality rate. And for women the figure jumps to 330 percent. Women have a smaller liver that metabolizes alcohol less efficiently.

Readers who wish to learn more about alcohol consumption should read *How Much Is Too Much* by Leonard Gross, published by Random House.

Does Alcohol Have Medicinal Value

How about some good news for a change? Let's forget, for a moment, the threat of nuclear war and the Salt II negotiations. Or inflation that governments can no longer control. Or the energy crunch which gets worse by the day. Rather, let's explore the medicinal virtues of alcohol. Could it be that modern physicians have sadly neglected this drug in an age of tranquilizers? Is it a sensible medication following surgery? Maybe even useful in cases of snakebite?

Alcoholic beverages have been prescribed by doctors for thousands of years. Alcohol is one of the oldest drugs known to man. Such a long-standing endorsement should alert today's physicians to its current possibilities.

Can alcohol be useful in treating one of the nation's greatest killers, cardiovascular disease? Some doctors are convinced it can play a worthwhile role. For example, Dr. Masters reported in 1937 in the *Journal of the American Medical Association* that the regular use of alcohol helped prevent coronary artery disease. This problem is less frequent in countries where wine is a part of the everyday diet. This same doctor, and others, also presented evidence that alcohol had a deterrent action in the development of atherosclerosis.

Alcohol can also be useful in relieving an attack of angina. Nitroglycerine and other modern drugs are better, but if they're not available, alcohol can relieve the pain. Moreover, some doctors have advised the use of either beer or wine in the prevention of such attacks.

Should you reach for the bottle to treat infection? It's been claimed that wine is of substantial value in the prevention of typhoid fever, cholera, and other bowel infections. But it may be the substitution of wine for contaminated water that is the contributing factor.

Few would disagree that alcohol is a useful adjunct when treating the common cold. Eight ounces of wine or 3 ounces of liquor rapidly dilate the peripheral blood vessels. This helps the induction of sweating, with resultant heat loss, lowering the body temperature. There's no doubt wine or liquor improve the psyche and induce drowsiness and a desire for sleep. Making disease more bearable is one of the prime functions of alcohol. And there is no better time to utilize this benefit than in older patients.

I think that North American morality keeps many physicians from recommending alcoholic beverages to patients. Consider the tens of thousands of arthritic patients who are rarely free from pain. Aspirin is still their best source of relief, but a drink or two during the day might do much to brighten their lives.

Harlow Brooks, a very wise physician, once said, "Either as a food, as a medicine, or for its comfort-giving qualities, alcohol properly administered is one of the greatest blessings of old age." And Canada's most distinguished doctor, Sir William Osler, aptly described it as "the milk of old age."

Today there's an overpowering tendency for doctors to prescribe tranquilizers to the aging. In my opinion, moderate alcohol consumption would be more effective, less troublesome, and a kindness to these patients.

What about its use following surgery? Doctors tend to forget the fear and apprehension that accompanies an operation, both before and after. They forget that many patients are accustomed to a drink before lunch or dinner. I don't think it's sensible to cut off a patient's customary glass of wine or eliminate his Scotch and soda at this time. I'm convinced we could reduce the need for pain-killing drugs a few days after surgery if we added alcohol to the post-operative routine of some patients.

Dr. Alhausen and his associates drove home an important point in 1960. Patients who have had part of all of the stomach removed often suffer from the malabsorption syndrome. There is loss of appetite, diarrhea, indigestion, weight loss, and pain. Alhausen discovered that the absorption of food could be restored in most cases by adding a dry, white table wine to the meal.

In Toronto's Sunnybrook Hospital is the Boar's Head, an English pub where patients can go to have a beer or two and ease mental and physical suffering. Sheila, the barmaid, is often more effective in treating illness than drugs or physicians. My research at the Boar's Head prompted me to conduct another study. Why not give surgical patients the option of one alcoholic drink before meals? Doctors tend to forget the apprehension of patients before and after surgery. A small amount of alcohol might ease some of that tension.

How do patients react to this choice? Some give me a skeptical glance and retort, "You're pulling my leg. It'll be a frosty morning before we're given a martini in the hospital." Others reply, "That would be great! I enjoy a glass of wine before dinner. I wonder why it's taken surgeons 2,000 years to suggest it."

But as with any research project, I encountered minor obstacles. For instance, many patients like the idea, but remarked, "Won't the nursing staff think I'm an alcoholic if you order a drink before meals?" There was an easy way around this fear. Patients were subsequently told that the nurses realized I was conducting a study. This gave the order an aura of respectability. Who wouldn't like to aid research by having a rum and coke or mint julep before dinner?

Another obstacle was also easily overcome. Hospitals can't operate a bar service, so the patient's family must be responsible for providing whatever beverage is desired. This is left at the nursing station along with physician's orders that it be served before mealtime.

What were the results? They followed a very consistent pattern. As you would expect, none of the patients asked for a drink on the first post-operative day. But by the second or third day it was welcome. Many stated that it helped to relieve the boredom and post-operative blues. They were more relaxed and slept better at night. And having a drink made them feel they would soon be home.

There was an interesting psychological reaction. The initial group of patients were only informed of this option during the early post-operative days. A more recent group were told prior to the surgery. This had an even better effect. One patient summed it up. She said, "Telling me I could have a drink after hysterectomy took away my fears. I thought you would never suggest it if I was going to be in serious trouble. I entered the hospital with more reassurance."

Would I continue this practice? You bet I would. I'm convinced it's sound medicine for patients. Alcohol is one of the oldest drugs known to man. Used in moderation it is a useful adjunct to medical care. One drink before mealtime will be part of my routine post-operative orders for those patients who wish it.

Why don't all hospitals have a "happy hour" then? It's because doctors, hospitals, and the general public are very inconsistent about morality. A bottle of beer is acceptable at the local bar. But walk into a hospital with some beer or a flask of whiskey and everyone thinks you're an alcoholic, that it's impossible for you to do without a drink for even a few days. Very few people would give you the benefit of the doubt. Yet you can walk into any hospital with a carton of cigarettes and smoke them continually. Or day after day devour tranquilizers, sleeping pills, and laxatives without being accused of addiction.

So far, Lady Luck has saved me from the surgeon's scalpel. But should my fortunes change, I'll practice what I preach. I'll arrive at the hospital with a small flask of rum. It will have "Research Study" stamped on the side. Hopefully that will give it an aura of respectability. It might also provide a good night's sleep without the side effects of sedatives and painkillers.

Can I Have a Scotch and Soda with This Pill?

"Can I take a Scotch and soda with this pill?" a newspaper editor recently asked me. The reply was an emphatic NO. It was a dangerous combination, and I have a practical aversion to losing editors. Imagine all the possible combinations of medicine and alcohol. We live in an over-medicated society, and it's the rare person who never takes an alcoholic drink. So what did I tell my editor? I told him about four Montana residents and their experience with beer.

Sir William Osler, the famous clinician, once remarked that, "A desire to take medicine is perhaps the great feature that distinguishes man from the other animals." In Osler's day there were fewer drugs. Today of the 100 most commonly used drugs about half contain at least one ingredient that reacts badly with alcohol. That's why in 1981, 50,000 North Americans who consumed alcohol while taking drugs were admitted to hospital emergency departments. More than 2,500 died from this combination.

Alcohol can affect drugs in several ways. The body's enzyme system gradually removes medicine from circulation. Alcohol slows down enzyme activity, causing a greater build-up of the drug in the body. Or it may increase absorption of drugs from the intestines, or dissolve the coating of time-release pills, giving a sudden dose of medication to the body.

People who are taking sedatives such as Phenobarbital or tranquilizers like Valium or Thorazine must cast a wary eye at their favorite bottle of Scotch. Alcohol and these drugs both depress the central nervous system. The additive effects can be lethal. For instance, Scotch and soda added to Phenobarbital means just half as much of this drug can kill you.

The body gets a double whammy in other ways. For instance many Canadians are taking anticoagulants or aspirin to help thin the blood. Add alcohol to these and too much thinning may occur, causing serious bleeding.

Alcohol is also bad news to that new diabetic who is being diagnosed every 60 seconds in North America. Some of these patients will need insulin, others oral agents such as orinase or diabenese, medications that lower blood sugar. Add Scotch and soda and a sharp drop in blood sugar level may cause sweating, pallor, weakness, dizziness, headache, palpitation of the heart, and fainting.

Be cautious of Scotch and soda if you're a heart patient. I'd agree a shot of brandy or favorite alcoholic drink is helpful if you suffer a heart spasm. But if you've reached for a nitroglycerine tablet to ease the coronary pain, stay away from any form of alcohol. The mixture can precipitate too much relaxation of blood vessels, triggering in turn low blood pressure and fainting.

Don't forget the other side of the coin—how ingested drugs affect the metabolism of alcohol. Under normal conditions your Scotch is oxidized to acetaldehyde and then to acetate. In 1937 Dr. E.E. Williams of Naugatuck, Connecticut, made a shrewd observation. Noting that rubber workers exposed to carbon disulfide developed an intolerance of alcohol, he suggested in the *Journal of the American Medical Association* that this phenomenon be used as a cure for alcoholism. But no one listened.

Disulfiram (antibuse) was developed 11 years later by Danish researchers. This drug prevents the normal breakdown of alcohol in the blood. The resulting high level of acetaldehyde causes flushing, sweating, shortness of breath, a rapid heart rate, nausea, and vomiting. It keeps some alcoholics honest. Other drugs can cause this antibuse-like reaction. The antibiotic chloromycetin; griseofulvin, a fungicide; and flagyl, used to treat trichomonas, a common vaginal infection, all possess this capability. The blood sugar regulators, orinase and diabenese, can also interfere with the metabolism of alcohol, causing a mild flushing.

The *New England Journal of Medicine* reports on four Montana residents who had picked and eaten wild mushrooms. The next day they were rushed to hospital after they had each consumed a bottle of beer. Their faces were flushed and they complained of a metallic taste in their mouths. It was followed quickly by numbness of the extremities, palpitation, nausea, and vomiting. They were sure it wasn't the result of mushrooms. Others had taken them without ill effects. But the doctors soon discovered that the others had not drunk beer.

These patients were simply unlucky. They had picked mushrooms that, eaten alone, would have had no toxic effects. But alcohol consumed even several hours later triggered a violent reaction. Why? Because antibuse is present in this particular type of mushroom.

The moral is, think twice before you mix drugs and alcohol. And if you like beer with mushrooms, make sure it's not the species *Coprinus atramentarius*!

Hangovers

We'd all like to escape hangovers, but most of us are laboring under misconceptions about expensive liquors. We're often buying the wrong wine, ignoring bottle corks, and we've never heard about chemical cogeners. That's partly why some of us can look forward to the wasteful morning-after debacle.

That last one for the road means agony for many. Excess alcohol consumption relaxes the muscles surrounding blood vessels in the brain. The engorged vessels in turn stretch nerve endings, and the hangover has begun.

But many don't know that the non-alcoholic substances called cogeners have the most effect on cranial blood vessels. Liquor companies use these additives to give color, flavor, and aroma to spirits and wines.

Dr. Gaston Pawan of Middlesex Hospital in London, England, recently conducted a very practical experiment. He had no trouble getting volunteers. He invited groups of men to weekly drinking sessions in a friend's apartment. They were served a meal and then festivities began. The men drank a pint of liquor, a different one each week. They left slightly inebriated and the next day reported on their hangovers. Dr. Pawan then rated the various drinks.

He found that brandy had the highest hangover rating. Red wine was a close second. It was followed by dark rum, sherry, Scotch, whiskey, beer, white wine, gin, and vodka. The popular U.S. drink, bourbon, wasn't tested, but it has a notorious reputation for producing a hangover. Dr. Pawan then gave the volunteers the same drinks but with cogeners removed by filtration. The men all reported fewer side effects.

This experiment suggests that the wealthy must have the worst hangovers. The oldest and most expensive drinks like bourbon and brandy are aged for some time in wooden barrels. During the aging process they absorb large amounts of cogeners from the wood. It also means that the Russians are one up on us. They have the ideal drink. Vodka is colorless, tasteless, and almost odorless. Minus most of the cogeners, it's little more than an unflavored ethyl alcohol and water.

What about wine, that sweet nectar of the gods? Luckily for wine lovers it contains smaller amounts of cogeners. But the color and price of wines do make a difference. Red wines are richly endowed with histamine, the substance manufactured by the body that triggers allergic reactions. Vintage wines from Burgundy may have 10 times as much as other reds, and 15 times the quantity of white wines. If your nose becomes congested after drinking red wine, it's due to the histamine content.

Do expensive wines, like costly liquors, cause a greater hangover? "Not so," says Dr. Pawan. Vintage wines contain fewer cogeners and are less likely to set the head throbbing.

Fortunately in these depressed financial times Dr. Pawan has a practical suggestion. It's possible to take some of the headache out of cheaper wines by removing the cork several hours before consumption. This allows the wine to breathe. In the process of breathing, cogeners evaporate more quickly than the alcohol.

But suppose you've done all the wrong things? What is the best way to treat a hangover? Contrary to folklore, another drink won't help. You'll simply bruise the brain a second time. And forget the raw eggs and Worcestershire sauce routine. This just invites the added problem of an upset stomach.

Aspirin and cold compresses help to constrict the brain's engorged vessels. Caffeine in black coffee or tea also aids in shrinking these vessels. And the sooner you rid your system of remaining alcohol the better.

The best treatment is to take fructose, one of the common sugars. Fructose increases the rate at which the body breaks down alcohol into innocent chemicals. Tomato juice, honey, apples, or grapes, in either liquid or solid form, have a high fructose content.

Then combat dehydration. Alcohol stimulates the kidneys, depleting the body of several nutrients. Salt is an important one. Various packaged broths will correct this situation as they contain salt and provide nourishment.

Before partying take a fructose drink to speed up the metabolism of alcohol. Then line the stomach with high-protein snacks such as milk, cheese, and meat to help prevent stomach irritation. Later take drinks with a fructose mix or a carbonated base like soda or quinine water.

Remember that some of the hangover may also be due to smoke inhalation. Move to a well-ventilated area, or go outside for some fresh air. Above all, be moderate. Euripides said in 300 B.C., "Enough is abundance to the wise." Things haven't changed.

8
General Surgery

Surgery and the Family Doctor

To stay healthy today it's necessary to keep a sense of humor. Without it you're more likely to develop ulcers, hypertension, and a sour personality. So a few days ago I followed my own advice and had a good laugh. My secretary told me a funny story about one of our delinquent accounts. It's a perfect example of what's happening to the practice of medicine. And how patients get into trouble by underestimating their family doctors.

My office had sent several bills to a patient with no result. Finally a call was made to enquire why no payment was forthcoming. The patient was very specific. She said, "I refuse to pay for that consultation. Why should I? The doctor didn't tell me anything different from my own family physician."

It seemed she would only pay for a new, exotic diagnosis of her problem. I had to prove her own doctor wrong, or at least raise some objection to his treatment. Then she would have considered my bill legitimate.

Luckily most patients think more logically. But there is an increasing tendency in North America to discount the family physician and place total faith in the infallibility of the specialist. Sometimes it should be the other way around. In some situations the family doctor is worth a cartload of super-specialists.

Consider this scenario. One morning I walked into the hospital recovery room. Several doctors were crowded around a patient on a stretcher. It was obvious they thought something was wrong. The patient's breathing, following a thyroid operation, was very labored.

Several speedy consultations had been arranged. An ear, nose, and throat specialist was convinced an emergency tracheotomy should be performed immediately. Two other surgeons agreed. Without an emergency airway the patient would soon suffocate.

Preparations were quickly made for surgery. But just as they were about to wheel the patient away, the family doctor arrived on the scene. The assembled consultants told him what they intended to do. He politely heard them out and listened to his patient's breathing.

Calmly and slowly he remarked, "Hell, I've known Herb for 20 years and he always breathes that way! He doesn't need a tracheotomy any more than the rest of us." The surgeons were not convinced but reluctantly agreed to delay the operation.

So, who was right? Later that day Herb was sitting up in bed, joking with his doctors, and still breathing heavily. He'll never know how close he came to having a needless operation. Fortunately he had a family doctor who was endowed with common sense. And one who possessed the intestinal fortitude to tell the specialists they were wrong.

The advantage of the family doctor is a long-term association with the patient and often a knowledge of family history. It is a current misconception, and a risky one, that the general practitioner knows less than a specialist.

During my training as a surgeon, I worked one summer as a general practitioner in La Mal Baie, Quebec. I lost count of the number of times an elderly French Canadian family doctor pulled me out of difficult situations. He was a very wise and kindly physician who performed a greater service to local families than a cartload of specialists could.

Specialists choose to work in a narrow field of medicine. They are expert in that field, but cannot know all the ramifications of a family's inherited health problems. This is where the referring practitioner excels and is invaluable.

What would I do if I became seriously ill? Like anyone else I'd like to be seen by the best doctors available. I might need super-specialists to treat my problem. But I've requested one condition under such circumstances. I'd want a family doctor to participate in the program of treatment.

When more than one specialist is involved, there can be disagreement about the proper course of action. That's when the common sense and sound judgment of a good family physician can separate the wheat from the chaff. The patient who refused to pay my bill doesn't know how lucky she is to have a good family doctor.

How Do You Choose a Surgeon?

"Wow!" my secretary exclaimed when she examined my car repair bill. "They've done it to you again! They know you're an easy mark and they load on the charges. I wouldn't pay it." Was she right? Did I have an honest car mechanic? Or one that was hoping to retire early in Florida? I admit I've met my Waterloo when it comes to auto mechanics. So let's make a deal. I'll tell you a foolproof way to find a capable surgeon. Will a reader reciprocate and give me the inside story on mechanics?

I have the easier assignment, because people labor under a misconception that the medical profession is a tightly closed circle. That doctors close ranks to protect one another. That some surgeons are arrogant egomaniacs. And unless you're a member of the group, there's no discussion of skills and abilities. So how could a lay person ever hope to search out the good surgeon from one who is all thumbs?

There's no denying some of these criticisms. We all know people who believe they can walk on water. The tendency to shelter medical colleagues who should have stopped operating years ago goes back to the beginnings of surgery. But none of these facts should have any bearing on the search for a capable surgeon.

What is the trick? Remember that there is a difference between surgeons and car mechanics. Surgeons always work with an audience. This visibility makes them vulnerable to criticism. Assistants, nurses, and anesthetists are subconsciously grading surgeons at each operation. This is what makes my assignment so easy. To find a first-class surgeon, you have to find a nurse.

Some readers will say, "That's not easy. We just moved and don't know a nurse. Or, "Nurses would never give me a name." Or, "It's unethical to ask a nurse." None of these excuses holds water. It's rare that a friend, next-door-neighbor or employer doesn't know a nurse. Or is unwilling to provide you with an introduction.

Scrub nurses who work in surgery day after day are the best guides to a first-class surgeon. But if your contact happens to work in the nursery, accept her advice anyway. It's easy for her to obtain information from a surgical nurse.

What about the family doctor? Can you trust his opinion when he suggests a surgeon? When I asked this question of a friend who's a medical university professor, he wasn't enthusiastic. He remarked, "Some GPs are not tuned in to surgery. They often have favorite surgeons for other than medical reasons. I'd be concerned that they might recommend their golfing buddy."

The professor may be partly right. If I moved to a new location, I'd place greater trust in a referral from a scrub nurse. But if a trusted family physician made a recommendation, I'd have no hesitation in accepting his opinion.

Many people believe all this advice is unnecessary—that all surgeons are qualified these days. That we've progressed since the horse-and-buggy days. That hospitals remove incompetent surgeons immediately. And that medical and government agencies are constant watchdogs over surgical practices.

This all sounds fine in theory. There's no doubt the practice of medicine has come a long way. But regulations are never the entire answer. Some doctors can pass written examinations, but they should never have chosen surgery as their specialty. It's unrealistic to assume that all surgeons have the same ability. One doesn't assume that of plumbers, pilots, engineers, or politicians.

Beware of other common fallacies. Don't decide on a friend's surgeon just because he is good looking and your friend survived the surgery. Don't accept the advice of a next-door-neighbor or employer. These individuals may believe they know who's who in surgery. But their decision is often based on hearsay evidence. The scrub nurse makes hers on daily performance. And never judge a surgeon by his bedside manner. I'd have Dracula remove my gallbladder if his skill in the operating room was the best in town.

Regrettably there are no scrub nurses watching car mechanics. But if someone knows a way of rating them I hope he'll let me know. I'm getting awfully tired of hearing my secretary say, "Wow! You've been taken again!"

Why the Rich Get Better Surgical Care

Scott Fitzgerald once remarked to Ernest Hemingway that the rich were different. "Yes, Scott," Hemingway replied, "they have more money." He could also have added that they usually get the best surgical care. Most people are operated on by quite adequate surgeons who have the right diplomas. Yet being adequate is not good enough for the rich or for doctors. These two groups want the best ones in town. If you have similar views, this article will show you how to end up with the same top surgeons.

One morning when I was promoting my book *The Doctor Game* I found myself in Saskatoon. I thought it would be another day of the same type of interviews, but the local radio station had done their homework well. As I sat down before the microphone, I noticed two interviewers instead of the usual one. I was informed that the extra guest was an executive from the Saskatchewan Medical Association and, like Mary Queen of Scots, I quickly surmised that I was about to get my head chopped off quite early in the morning.

This doctor politely told me and the listening audience that there were some worthwhile things in the book, but like any good debater he was also setting me up for the kill. Eventually he made his thrust. He assured all the listeners that if either of us should suddenly need our gallbladder removed in Saskatoon there wasn't any need for the book. Why? Because all the surgeons in Saskatoon were well-qualified ones. We could literally take our pick and it wouldn't matter who finally picked up the scalpel.

In one way he was right. Most likely on any given day all the surgeons in Saskatoon could remove the same appendix or gallbladder with the same final results. So, Gifford-Jones, why don't you pack your bag and move on to the next town, where they're not smart enough to have you face a knowledgeable executive from the SMA?

One reason I didn't quickly fold my tent was because it was about 20° below zero outside and I was still thawing out. Besides there's more to surgery than one gallbladder and one given day. Then there was also that old feeling that some doctors tend to talk out of the corners of their mouths. This "all is well" talk may fool some people—like, maybe, those who are awfully proud of Saskatoon. However, I'm sure it didn't persuade any of the financially successful citizens of that city. None of them became rich by shutting their eyes and rolling the dice on business deals, and I imagine many of them smiled when it came over the radio.

In Saskatoon, or any other city, there is only one way I'd accept any surgeon without question. I'd have to be brought to the hospital unconscious! To say that all surgeons are of equal competence is naive, childish, and deceptive advice, and there is not one doctor in Saskatoon who would be willing to throw a dart at the list to pick out his surgeon.

How do the rich get superior surgical care? A Japanese proverb states, "Money has no ears, but it hears." Wealthy people simply have easy access to sources that automatically point them in the right direction. Sometimes the well-to-do find out "who's who" while playing a round of golf with one of the doctors. It's easy to say, "Art, the family doctor tells me I need an operation. He's given me four names, but confidentially who is the best?"

The rich, however, are not infallible. Sometimes they commit the same errors as people of more moderate means. They, too, take the advice of non-medical social contacts who think they know "who's who" in surgery. Yet operating room nurses, who are in daily contact with the best, and the worst, would laugh at their choice.

How does the average person keep pace with the wealthy and end up with one of the grade A surgeons in the community? For one thing, you have to keep your feet on the ground with health insurance. Most people now have easy access to surgical care, and this tends to give an overall feeling of complacency and security but, remember, it's the individual surgeon who makes the incision—not the government plan.

People of modest means don't play golf with the top surgeons, but everyone can obtain inside information about surgeons with a minimum of effort. The prime advice is, "Get to a nurse," ideally an operating room scrub nurse. She knows the good technicians from the diddlers, but other nurses can still get this information for you. So can switchboard operators, secretaries, laboratory technicians, and boiler room workers. The hospital grapevine is usually right on. Make sure that you use it when picking out a surgeon.

Remember, too, that the rich and doctors also have one thing in common. They would both head the list of the nation's top hypochondriacs. After all, the rich have a lot to lose by leaving this planet, and doctors hate to pack their bags prematurely, just on general principles. These two groups are, therefore, very careful about their own bodies and check and double-check before submitting to a particular surgeon. It's for this reason that the Saskatoon philosophy is politically safe for public consumption, but it doesn't hold water. It's a "do as I say, not as I do" approach.

Sophocles in 450 B.C. wrote, "Money lays waste cities; it sets men to roaming from home; it seduces and corrupts honest men and turns virtue to baseness; it teaches villany and impiety." Nowadays Sophocles would still be right on, but he could add that moneyed people get better care because they invariably find out "who's who" in surgery. If it's a sound approach for the rich, it's also a wise move for others.

Be Careful Where Super-Surgery Is Done

A reader living in a city of 100,000 people writes, "One of the local surgeons has previously removed my gallbladder and repaired a hernia. Now at 70 years of age I have a blocked artery in one leg. The surgeon has advised a bypass operation to circumvent the obstruction and ease the pain. He enjoys an excellent local reputation and the other operations have gone well. But I understand this is a very major type of surgery and my wife wants me to obtain another opinion. Would this be a wise move?"

This letter brings up a pertinent question. In effect it asks whether surgeons in a small city should do super-surgery. Or should these cases be channeled to a university teaching hospital where such procedures are done on a regular basis? It's a difficult question to answer, but some specific guidelines might help.

Just where major surgery ends and super-surgery begins is tough to pin-point in all cases. Certainly transplanting a heart or kidney is in the super-surgery category. The bypass operation in which a graft shunts blood around an obstruction may not be as dramatic. But it's still very complex surgery and can be an extremely tedious undertaking for doctors who are tackling it only occasionally.

Canadians are more protected from super-surgery than Americans. It would be impossible for Canadians to have cardiac surgery in a small community hospital; the government refuses to purchase equipment for a hospital that does not have proper staff and back-up facilities.

In the U.S. any hospital can carry out these procedures if they can afford the expensive setup and have doctors on staff willing to undertake the surgery. That's why statistics show some small hospitals in that country with mortality rates for heart surgery that are 3 to 10 times those of well-qualified university centers.

But certain operations, like bypassing a clogged artery, can be performed with less equipment. This exposes some Canadians to a potentially dangerous trap.

Odd as it may seem, today's better-trained surgeons in a community raise some problems that were not present in past years. The older generation of surgeons were never exposed to vascular techniques. Consequently it never entered their minds to attempt them. Many recent graduates have spent time working with vascular surgeons during their training. Some of these doctors performed a reasonable number of such operations prior to starting practice. When they left the university hospital, they had every hope of continuing to do so.

One major problem confronts them. Vascular procedures are not as common as hernias, gallbladders, and hemorrhoid operations. So in the average Canadian community young doctors end up doing these more frequent procedures. These surgeons may be very capable technicians and develop a large referring practice. Then somewhere along the line they once again get involved with vascular work. A sudden emergency may arise and there's no time to refer the patient to another hospital. Or they may gradually slip back into this work as they encounter problems.

But being a now-and-then vascular surgeon can be a potentially dangerous game. Neither the surgeon nor the operating room scrub nurses ever get into high gear. Surgeons, like plumbers, must do the same thing over and over to develop and maintain skills.

What should the patient do? It's in this and so many other situations that the family doctor is worth his weight in gold. He will only receive a few dollars for his advice. But in steering you away from a hazardous situation he may save your life.

A good family physician will have several questions in mind when making a decision. He will ask whether the doctor limits his work to this type of surgery. And if so, is he performing several cases a week? Has he had good training? Would he refer a member of his own family to this surgeon?

I think most family doctors share my view. They want good results for their patients. The best guarantee is to refer them to a full-time vascular surgeon. It's the route doctors would follow with their own families.

Is an Older Surgeon a Safe Surgeon?

Mr. E.L. of Montreal writes, "I've been reading your column for the past year and would like your advice. An older surgeon says my gallbladder should be removed. He's about 65 and was recommended by my family doctor. Would you consider doing a column on this topic? Maybe other readers have wondered if it's safe to have their operation done by an older man."

Another person, Mrs. D.C. of Winnipeg, questions. "I know you are against general practitioners performing surgery, but when do you believe that qualified surgeons should call it a day? Do hospitals have controls that protect patients from this problem? My husband needs an operation and I would prefer to see it carried out by a younger surgeon. I'd appreciate your comments."

These two letters bring up the age-old question of when aging surgeons should put down the scalpel. It can be an important issue, because some elderly surgeons sooner or later become a hazard to the public. What should you do if you're presented with this problem?

Surgeons, like sports stars, also reach their peak at a certain age, but there is a big difference between these two groups. The aging hockey player who is becoming a shadow of his former self can't hide his deficiencies from the public. The cold, critical eye of the TV camera eventually picks him out, and the former cheers of the crowd also change to boos. Some players quickly hear these early cries and hang up their skates. But if they do have a deaf ear to these calls, there is one other major control over professional players. They come under the eagle eye of their coaches, who have no desire to either lose games or their jobs.

Surgeons, on the other hand, are not subjected to the weekly scrutiny of television, and most are their own managers. Some faltering surgeons can therefore present a danger to patients if they have a never-give-up attitude and want to continue on to the bitter end. They can also cause a somewhat perplexing problem for their own colleagues.

There are few sadder sights in an operating room than the gradual demise of a surgeon who used to be tops in his field. Some continue on because of an intense devotion to their work. Others have too much ingrained egomania to lay down the scalpel. Still others in these days of increasing inflation have insufficient funds to retire.

But regardless of the reason, their colleagues rarely take them aside and politely ask them to quit. It's always an embarrasing situation, so nearly everyone skirts around the problem and hopes they'll retire on their own initiative. Moreover, during my years of surgery I've never witnessed any official from our licensing bodies observing a surgeon whose hands and eyesight are failing. In practice it therefore becomes a problem for that particular hospital, and most take the position of "once a surgeon always a surgeon." Few hospitals have mandatory ages for retirement.

What should patients do if they find themselves in the hands of a 65-year-old surgeon? First of all, don't panic and automatically assume he's lost his golden touch. I know some senior surgeons who can still operate rings around their junior colleagues. They were always magnificent technicians, and age hasn't removed this skill.

Remember, too, that some older surgeons possess the characteristics of good wine. They're mature, seasoned operators with thousands of cases behind them, and they have two advantages over those who are still in knee pants. Before the surgery you have a greater chance of getting a balanced opinion from him as to the need of the operation. Second, if he encounters an unexpected problem once the incision has been made, he can draw on years of experience to deal with it in the most satisfactory way. I would have no hesitation being wheeled into surgery by a senior surgeon as long as I knew he still had capable hands and an alert brain.

But how does the person on the street separate the top surgeons from the diddlers? If you've been referred to him by the family doctor that is usually a good recommendation. They have no desire to spend three hours assisting at an operation that should be done in half the time, and they also like to see their patients end up with good results. Yet if this question continues to cause concern, ask your general practitioner about it. After all, if you can't communicate with him on such matters, you've got the wrong doctor.

But never, never listen to gossip because, like hot tips on the stock market, it can give you the wrong information. So if you want to check up on a senior surgeon ask someone who is in the know. Earlier I advised you to seek the opinion of hospital "insiders," as they either know or can easily find out who has the best hands. Nurses are the prime insiders, and you should always endeavor to locate one. But if I lived next door to the boiler room attendant, I'd still sleep well if his enquiries told me that a 65-year-old surgeon was still the best one in town for that particular operation.

Lastly, remember that age is only one way to gage a surgeon, and that there are good and bad ones in every age bracket. There obviously comes a time when advancing years catch up with the best of them, but at 65 some surgeons do not need to be put out to pasture.

Dog Collars Could Help Stop Anesthetic Fatalities

How safe is it to have an anesthetic in 1984? Most readers never ask this question until a major anesthetic accident hits the headlines. Then my mail is full of letters from concerned patients who are about to have an operation. Why do these accidents occur? And how could a dog collar prevent such disasters?

Dr. H.K. Beecher, professor of anesthesia at Harvard, reported in 1954 on a study of 600,000 anesthetics given at 10 U.S. hospitals. His conclusion? Patients had 1 chance in 95 of dying from the disease that brought them to the hospital. And 1 chance in 2,680 of succumbing because of anesthesia.

Another study in Australia between 1960 and 1968 revealed that anesthetists have an average of one anesthetic death during their lifetime of medical practice, and an average of 4.3 near fatalities for every one of these deaths.

The British Association of Anesthetists conducted a study on all the surgical deaths that occurred in England, Scotland, and Wales during 1979. Three million anesthetics had been given that year. They concluded that 300 fatalities were directly related to the anesthesia. A further 600 were strongly linked but not completely due to the anesthetic complication. The risk of dying from an anesthetic is therefore about 1 chance in 10,000. A French survey of 200,000 anesthetics reached similar conclusions.

What exactly causes these deaths? The British study showed that faulty anesthetic technique was responsible for 43 percent of the deaths and the incorrect use of anesthetic agents caused 17 percent of the fatalities.

Drs. J.B. Cooper and R.S. Newbower in 1984 reported in the *American Journal of Anesthesiology* on 1,089 preventable accidents. The troubles most often encountered were disconnection of the anesthetic circuit, loss of the gas supply, errors in administering drugs, or the unexpected reaction of the patient to the anesthetic agents. Other studies cite the failure of anesthetists to maintain an adequate airway, failure to maintain ventilation, and the inability of the doctor to either recognize or cope with the problem during surgery. Just 4 percent of serious incidents are due to equipment failure.

Patients should be reassured that the number of anesthetic deaths have decreased over the years. But there's a rather disturbing fact: the causes of death remain the same. Human error continues to be the major problem.

Why do machines have a better track record than humans? A prime reason is that anesthetic machines stay where they're supposed to be during the surgery, next to the patient. They never need to go to the bathroom. They never receive domestic calls from wives. They have no desire to telephone their stockbroker for the latest quotation on Quick Rich Mines. Nor do they read the latest bestseller at the operating table.

Doctors have a cardinal rule drummed into them during anesthesia training. Never, never abandon an unconscious patient without leaving a qualified substitute in charge. But there are still too many wandering anesthetists in this country. And I don't believe research has ever proved that they have smaller bladders than the rest of the population.

A frustrated surgeon once said to me, "I'd like to put a dog collar around the necks of my anesthetists and attach it to their machine." There's no doubt that some catastrophic accidents could be avoided if anesthetists were in constant attendance.

Can this problem be solved? It's not the patient's job to persuade the doctor to stay with her/him during the surgery. Patients have enough to worry about with an upcoming operation. And I'm convinced that doctors will never solve this matter themselves. They either play golf with their wandering colleague, or anesthetists simply ignore pleas to stop wandering to the telephone.

There's only one solution. Hospital boards should establish rules that anesthetists stay with their patients throughout surgery or lose their hospital privileges. Malpractice insurance companies should also inform anesthetists their company will not pay malpractice claims if it can be proven the doctor was absent during surgery.

Fortunately the majority of patients have the ever-watchful eye of a conscientious anesthetist. There are also few things in life where the odds are as good as 1 in 10,000. But we could improve these odds if the wandering anesthetist became past history.

How to Prepare for an Operation

What would God do if He were a surgeon? If the saying is true that God helps those who help themselves, He would refuse to operate on many of us. I'm sure He would tell us, "Respect your own God-given body and then I'll do what I can." Even a benevolent God might get fed up and throw up His hands in despair over some patients.

Consider the utter idiocy of this case. A 45-year-old woman underwent an operation for extensive vaginal repair. Her surgeon warned her repeatedly about the hazards of smoking and her persistent smoker's hack after this type of surgery. Ten days later she was rushed to hospital because of sudden postoperative hemorrhage. Incredibly, she was still smoking and coughing convulsively as she lay in a pool of blood in the emergency room. In this case speedy surgery stopped the bleeding.

But God must be tired of seeing the needless tragedy that strikes some families. During my final year of medical school a 45-year-old diabetic weighing 275 pounds was admitted to the Massachusetts General Hospital due to an acute gallbladder attack. A skilled surgeon removed the organ, but a lifetime of bad habits began slowly to take its toll.

The patient's diabetes was hard to control and the incision in the pendulous abdomen became infected. Shortly after, the man developed pneumonia, phlebitis, and blood clots in the lungs. Day after day his wife and children watched the complications multiply and his condition deteriorate. When he finally succumbed to overwhelming odds, his wife demanded of the professor, "Why did this happen to my husband? Why did you let him die? Couldn't something have been done to save his life?"

The professor listened sympathetically and patiently at first. But finally, because of pent-up frustration, he replied, "Look—God didn't kill your husband. Nor has he died because of fate or what this hospital has done. This death didn't just happen. Your husband killed himself. He'd been warned for years that it was essential to lose weight, stop smoking, and get more exercise. But this advice fell on deaf ears."

No doctor turns away a patient who has an acute surgical problem. But patients can't expect doctors to work miracles with surgery when they haven't given a tinker's damn about their bodies for years. I think God would agree it's time to issue an ultimatum to everyone. God and surgeons shouldn't attempt the impossible. And patients should be expected to help themselves by shaping up beforehand.

How can pre-operative patients shape up for an operation? Surgery, like tennis or football, demands some psychological preparation. A good start is to get rid of needless worries. Tell the doctor if you are overcome by a fear of not surviving the surgery. Or if you're concerned about post-operative pain. Or confused about which organs will be removed. And if you're apprehensive about the length of the incision, remember Abe Lincoln's remark. He was once asked, "How long should a man's leg be?" He replied, "Just long enough to reach the ground." Incisions, like legs, are just long enough to do the job safely.

Surgeons would need divine intervention to answer other questions. I recently examined a woman with a huge abdominal mass. It was impossible to know if the enlargement was due to a massive ovarian cyst, a benign fibroid, or a malignancy. Yet the patient demanded assurance that a hysterectomy wouldn't be done and that one ovary would be left in place. No surgeon can make that kind of guarantee until the abdomen is opened.

But the main thrust of preparation should be directed at good physical conditioning. Every year about 125 Americans die in commercial aviation accidents. But between 2,000 and 15,000 U.S. citizens have anesthetic deaths. Some of these tragedies could be prevented if patients tossed away cigarettes before an operation or made a genuine attempt to control and lose weight.

Trouble can also result when pre-operative patients don't inform the doctor of their medication. Water pills can deplete the body's potassium; low potassium combined with anesthesia increases the risks. Potent tranquilizers should be stopped several days prior to an operation. Inform the doctor if you're taking blood pressure pills, anti-glaucoma drops, or cortisone. And if you've disguised a glass eye from friends, don't hide it from the anesthetist. A glass eye that doesn't react to light could spell troubles if the anesthetist is not aware of it.

My advice is to be prepared for possible surgery all of the time. This means having a life-long respect for mind and body. It would give surgeons fewer grey hairs. Fewer families would be asking why post-operative complications occurred. And I'm sure God would be more willing to help those who help themselves.

Surgery and the Elderly

More and more people are becoming senior citizens. There will be an even larger number in the future. It means an increasing amount of surgery is being done for wear-and-tear problems. On the one hand, it's been a tremendous boon to be able to repair troublesome hernias and fallen wombs or add new spare parts to worn-out structures.

But whether or not the surgery should be done is often the $64 question. Some people rush into an operation that should not be done. Others endure annoyances for years that could be safely relieved by surgery. Are there some sensible guidelines that will help patients and their families decide on the proper course?

Unfortunately, some people immediately become pessimistic about elderly patients. Senior citizens have some very positive things going for them.

It's been said facetiously that you can't be too particular in picking out your parents. Most elderly people had parents who similarly went down the road a good distance. But sound, solid genes give people more than a long life. These patients frequently have more bounce in their step. It's a great help in pulling them through an operation.

During my years of surgical practice, I've formulated one strong impression about older patients. It's simply that many of them are tough. I've repeatedly seen them sail through an operation with less fuss and fuming than some patients in their 20s.

Aristotle made a cogent remark about them over 2,000 years ago. He said, "There are no boy philosophers." I think he hit it right on the head. Some elderly patients have a pretty sound outlook on life. This, too, stands them in good stead at the time of surgery.

I recall one 91-year-old patient who detected that I was concerned about her age. She had an early cancer, and it was imperative to do an operation. Jokingly she said to me, "Don't worry about me doctor. The worst thing that can happen to me is that I'll just die." Yet a few days after the surgery she was helping a 20-year-old in the same room who had less get-up and go.

In assessing the pros and cons of surgery at this age, it's important to be realistic. Do you have a genuine complaint? How much annoyance is it causing? Then check with the surgeon on the amount of risk. Don't forget to ask what are the chances of cure. Sometimes it's better to take a small risk than live with a troublesome problem. Several months ago I had a call from an internist. He had an 82-year-old woman with severe urinary incontinence. Otherwise she enjoyed good health. But now she had been forced to withdraw from her bridge club. It was the one thing she lived for, week after week. Now she had become despondent. He wondered if I would consider doing an operation.

This lady had a bona fide complaint. She also had a lot of zest for life. Now she's back with her old bridge cronies. The small risk was well worth the end result.

But sometimes the risk is too great and the results too questionable. Another elderly patient complained of intermittent claudication in one leg. The artery was partially blocked by arteriosclerosis. It meant that every hundred feet he had to stop for a minute to ease the pain. Yet it required a complicated operation to bypass the obstruction. Besides, the potential results were questionable in this case.

Luckily this man had gone to a cardiovascular surgeon noted for his good judgment. He advised against the operation. Several years later this patient was still around and had learned to live with his disability. It could have been a different story if an operation had been done.

Surgeons have to take extra care in preparing older patients for an operation. An underlying anemia may require a few weeks of treatment, or a diabetic problem may require time to be brought under better control. Failure to play it close to the chest may tip the scale the wrong way.

But patients and their family must realize that some things are virtually impossible to correct. Lungs that have been damaged by years of smoking can't be quickly repaired. Nor can the 250-pound patient suddenly win the battle against obesity. And some patients have to enter the operating room with blood pressures that are higher than the surgeon likes to see.

In these instances there is an increased risk to any operation. These patients are more likely to develop incisional hernias, infection, pneumonia, and phlebitis. Some of these people are their own worst enemies. So often I've seen patients with a chronic cough and post-operative temperature who nevertheless try to sneak a cigarette when you're not looking. Remember that it's only possible for doctors to be their brothers' keepers to a certain extent.

You should also bear in mind that there is a great difference between chronological and biological age. The patient who looks years younger than his age usually comes through the operation with flying colors. Another who looks 10 years older than his age has an increased chance of being headed for trouble.

Fancy tests are sometimes required to separate the good from the poor risk patients. But usually this isn't the case. Some 75-year-old patients jump on and off the examining table with relative ease. Just using your eyes should even tell the lay person they are good candidates for surgery.

Cataract Surgery

Is it advisable to have an operation to remove a cataract? Or is it wiser to live with the disability? In recent years tremendous advances have been made in cataract surgery. For some patients the results are miraculous. But others wish they had never consented to the procedure. This usually happens when patients fail to understand the implications of the operation.

Cataracts are the leading cause of partial blindness throughout the world. In Canada they're the leading cause of hospital admissions for eye surgery, and in North America over 200,000 cataract operations are performed every year.

Cataracts are opacities in the eye lens. They occur for various reasons. Some children are born with congenital cataracts. Others develop them when the mother has German measles early in pregnancy. Still others result from injury, diabetes, glaucoma, radiation, electric shock from lightning, or prolonged cortisone therapy. Ninety percent occur in elderly people.

The onset of a cataract produces a number of symptoms—perhaps a slow painless decrease in vision, or a rapid loss in sight and frequent changes of glasses. Some patients complain of fixed spots, glare from lights, or halos while driving at night. A loss of color vision or a yellowing is often experienced.

But there is one very characteristic symptom. Some patients get so-called "second sight." They're pleased to discover a rejuvenation of sight, making it possible to read without glasses.

People who develop cataracts should be aware of one point. These can cause a wide range of visual problems, which can vary from mild impairment to severe loss. But cataracts alone never result in total blindness.

Cataracts should not be removed merely because they're present. It's safer to postpone surgery until either work or activities are impaired. The timing for the operation therefore differs from one person to another.

Newspaper editors, doctors, and lawyers who must read thousands of words every week can't function without good vision. Others who are retired or who are not dependent on reading for enjoyment may not complain about a decrease in eyesight.

If cataracts are causing trouble, on the other hand, it's no longer necessary to delay surgery until they're mature. Luckily the complications of cataract surgery are small. There's only a 5 percent chance of post-operative problems. And just 1 chance in 5,000 that an eye will be lost to infection after surgery.

Why is a patient sometimes unhappy after a cataract is removed from one eye? The procedure involves removal of the lens. This means the eye loses its ability to focus on objects at varying distances. The full implications of this loss are hard to explain to patients. So people are sometimes shocked when they realize their vision has not been restored to normal.

The time-honored way to compensate for loss of the lens has been the adoption of thick glasses. Regrettably, this doesn't completely solve the problem. Objects in the central vision will be in focus with these glasses, but the peripheral vision remains distorted. There's also a loss of panoramic vision. And since objects are made 25 percent larger, they seem closer than they are. This causes difficulty in reaching for things or judging distances while walking down stairs.

There's another hazard. Since the eye after surgery sees everything 25 percent larger and the good eye records objects normal in size, the brain can't fuse these different images. Patients can never use both eyes to focus on objects. They must learn to use one eye until another cataract is removed to make both eyes equal. It's easy to see why some regret having one cataract removed if the other eye remains normal.

Luckily there is a way around this dilemma for 80 percent of patients, those who can learn to use contact lenses. These lenses reduce the change in size to 8 percent and the brain can accept this smaller disparity between eyes.

What does the future hold? Currently, in an increasing number of cases, ophthalmologists are inserting an artificial lens at the time of surgery. Long-term tolerance of the intraocular lens transplant is not yet known.

Is there any way to prevent cataracts? Recent medical literature states that vitamin E has proven effective in test-tube experiments. But as yet its effectiveness on the human eye has not been determined.

Coronary Bypass

Consider this nerve-wracking decision for a German surgeon in 1897. A 22-year-old gardener had been stabbed in the heart with a kitchen knife during a drunken brawl. Surgeons at that time believed it was madness to operate on the heart. But Ludwig Rehn decided nevertheless to open the patient's chest. He placed two silk stitches in the heart wound. To everybody's surprise, the patient survived. But it was the first time this type of surgery had been attempted. A year later Rehn presented a report on his surgical triumph at the International Congress of Surgeons in Berlin.

Rehn would be astounded at the progress in cardiac surgery in the last few decades. This past week I witnessed a superb team of cardiac surgeons at Toronto's Western Hospital performing a coronary bypass operation. For sheer drama there is no other surgery like it. To see a patient's chest open, the sternum parted, and the surgeon calmly holding the pulsing heart in his hands is a miracle in itself. It's a scene that would terrify a child, fascinate a philosopher, and send an artist scurrying for his brushes. This year over 125,000 bypass operations will be done in North America. Unless Canadians and Americans change their lifestyle drastically, more will be needed in future.

North America has become the atherosclerotic center of the world. We've achieved this dubious distinction by consuming garbage foods that produce garbage diseases like hardening of the arteries, diabetes, and hypertension.

Atherosclerosis, similar to a clogged drainpipe, decreases the flow of blood to the heart's muscle, causing anginal pain. The coronary bypass creates a detour so that blood gets past the blockage. It often cures the pain and may help to prevent a fatal myocardial infarction. But there is continuing debate as to whether this surgery actually prolongs life.

Two operating teams are required for this technique. One surgeon removes a long segment of the saphenous vein in the leg to act as the bypass graft. This vein is chosen for several reasons. It's the vein that is removed during varicose vein operations and, like the appendix, we can live without it. The vein is also close to the surface. And since it's the patient's own tissue, it eliminates the possibility of rejection by the body.

Another surgeon opens the chest through the sternum (breastbone) to expose the heart. The patient's circulatory system is then connected to a heart-lung machine. This apparatus has made cardiac surgery possible because surgeons cannot place delicate stitches in coronary vessels while the heart is beating. The heart-lung machine acts as a temporary pump for the heart and also functions as the patient's lungs.

The heart is put at rest by placing a plastic tube into its right chamber. This tube takes the oxygen-poor venous blood returning to the heart to the machine. As the blood travels through the machine it picks up a fresh supply of oxygen. Blood is then pumped back into the circulatory system by another tube inserted into the aorta, the main artery of the body.

The heart-lung machine also cools the blood to decrease body temperature. Lowering the metabolic needs of the heart and other tissues by this means puts them into a state of hibernation. This allows the surgeon about 90 minutes for the bypass operation. One end of the saphenous graft is connected to the aorta and the other end is stitched into the unblocked part of the coronary vessel.

The number of bypasses created in one operation is determined by the condition of the vessels. Usually three or four are required. But as many as 10 have been done in extreme cases. Once the grafts are completed, the surgeon allows the heart gradually to take over the work of the heart-lung machine.

Impending heart surgery always triggers an enormous emotional response from the patient and his or her family. It takes a hardy person not be fearful and apprehensive. But some patients also become angry that fate has dealt them this blow. This is particularly true if they have friends of the same age who have led a careless life but remain apparently free of trouble. For the thin, athletic, non-smoking person the sense of injustice becomes very obvious.

Ludwig Rehn would applaud the low mortality rate of the coronary bypass operation. Today 98 percent of patients survive the procedure when it's performed by a crack surgical team. Like a well-conducted orchestra, the technique is a joy to watch. But in less skilled hands the mortality rate can reach 15 percent.

Edward Gibbon, author of *The Decline and Fall of the Roman Empire*, remarked, "The winds and the waves are always on the side of the ablest navigator." This is also true for plumbers, TV repairmen, and cardiac surgeons.

Patients about to undergo cardiac surgery would be well advised to read *Open Heart Surgery* by Ina L. Yalof. It's published by Random House in both Canada and the U.S.

Preventing "Bone Disasters" in Children

Bad surgical results are hard to accept at any age, but they are particularly hard to swallow when they occur in young children. Moreover, some post-operative complications merely cause temporary inconvenience and worry, yet others result in a lifetime of tragedy, not only for the child, but also for despondent parents.

During the past year I've received several sad, probing letters from parents about their children. The general tone of these letters and the sequence of catastrophic events frequently followed a similar pattern, and many centered around orthopedic complications. Now they were asking how I could help them solve these difficulties once the damage had been done.

Regrettably some children are born with a club foot, too much curvature of the legs, an easily dislocated hip, or other bony abnormalities. Birth deformities always come as a terrible shock to parents, and it's understandable that they want them corrected at the earliest possible time. However, in preparing the stage for surgery parents must keep some basic facts in mind.

Orthopedic specialists are the surgical engineers of the operating room. Today, as in the past, they spend much of their time trying to reconstruct shattered bones resulting from automobile accidents and from a variety of other misfortunes. But now due to better techniques and new materials, they're also able to make new hip joints for arthritic patients and ease the pain of many other problems that occur in later life. At the other end of life's spectrum, they can also perform corrective operations on the deformed bones of young children.

Surgical engineers who wield the scalpel, however, are not as fortunate as engineers who use the slide-rule. If you're building a crane, you can throw around a lot of stresses and strains, add a few fancy equations, and usually end up with the right answer. Parents must realize that, although the scalpel normally does a good job, it is still not an exact science. Besides, orthopedic specialists are really "big plastic surgeons," and whether you're lifting a face or reconstructing a bone it's impossible to be sure of the final result.

One parent told me they had been informed that nothing could go wrong. Years later these words were still ringing in their ears after a child had undergone a series of operations in an endeavor to rectify a poor surgical result. Another parent sent a 10-page letter about how they had been intimidated by the haughty attitude of a surgeon who skirted around the possibility of complications. Yet their child had been operated on in several major hospitals as they tried to undo the complications of the first surgery.

Communication with your doctor is vital in every field of surgery, but it is absolutely essential when corrective operations are being performed on bone. I'm sure that most orthopedic surgeons are not naive enough to hand parents a written guarantee for an excellent result for their child. But if you ever run into one that does vouch for the perfect outcome, place him on the suspect list and get another opinion.

What about second opinions? Is it always a wise idea to obtain one even under the best of conditions? It would certainly be irresponsible for Gifford-Jones to send parents scurrying all over Canada to obtain additional advice for every birth deformity. Second opinions can be excess baggage for straightforward problems. Besides there are well-trained orthopedic surgeons in some small communities who are quite capable of handling many of these difficulties.

But let's consider the other side of the coin. Some problems that landed on my desk this past year might have been averted by an unbiased consultation. It could have stopped some operations from being done. Moreover, in the event of a complication developing, parents have the satisfaction of knowing they received the green light from more than one doctor. Lastly, remember that it always pays to be careful in assessing your own surgical problem. All the more reason to be doubly cautious in dealing with your child's difficulty.

Will an orthopedic surgeon resent a consultation and assume you're doubting his professional integrity? There is always a chance it will ruffle his fur a bit, but this also indicates you may be in the wrong office. A busy, seasoned surgeon with a balanced judgment welcomes another opinion, if for no other reason than for easing the parents' concern.

Several letters also had a recurring theme that is worth mentioning. Some parents wished they had never agreed to the surgery in the first place. They now realized that their child had been born with a relatively minor abnormality, but it had required a major operation in an attempt to correct it. The end result was worse than the original problem. Consequently, make certain that a small deformity can be rectified by a minor operation. If it needs a major procedure think twice about it. Striving for perfection is an admirable trait, yet it can also backfire on parents.

The best insurance in preventing "bone disasters" is getting into the hands of a top-drawer technical surgeon who has sound judgment and the ability to communicate the pros and cons of the surgery. Don't forget the advice I've given earlier on how to obtain inside information about the doctors in your area. Doing your homework this way will usually place your child in competent hands.

Tonsillectomy

A nagging doubt occurs routinely in thousands of homes. A doctor has suggested that a child needs a tonsillectomy. Today's informed parents now wonder whether the operation is truly needed. It's an important decision when about one in seven children undergoes such surgery, sometimes needlessly. But guidelines do exist that help parents to know when it's better to agree to an operation. Or to use antibiotics instead. Or at times to do nothing.

Tonsillectomy has always been under a cloud of suspicion. And for good reason. I reported several years ago that children in North America are 12 times more likely to have tonsils removed than children in Sweden. Also, wide variations occur in the number of tonsillectomies done in different parts of North America. It's impossible to justify regional differences on purely medical grounds. Too often tonsillectomies are done for financial reasons or, like circumcision, for almost ritualistic reasons.

Tonsillitis can be caused by either bacterial or viral infection. But the most common culprit is the beta hemolytic streptococcus germ. It's commonly referred to as "strep throat" and primarily strikes children under 10 years of age.

Today tonsillitis is looked on as a minor problem. But before antibiotics were available, this infection often initiated middle ear infections, glomerulonephritis, acute kidney inflammation, or rheumatic fever that caused swelling of the joints.

Even now it's still hard to remove the element of emotionalism from this operation. Some die-hards preach that all infected tonsils must be removed. Still others violently oppose the operation except under extreme circumstances. Small wonder that parents become confused as to who is right.

Practically every child with a sore throat also has inflamed and enlarged tonsils. The majority of throat infections are picked up at school. These children should initially be treated with antibiotics; penicillin remains the drug of choice unless the child is sensitive to this medication. But parents must realize that, once started, penicillin or any other antibiotic must be continued for 10 days. Failure to do so may not eradicate the streptococcus germ.

Remember, too, that not every sore throat needs antibiotics. The inflamed throat may be the result of a viral infection. Penicillin has no effect on a virus. Besides, most cases of sore throat and tonsillitis can still be cured by tincture of time and throat gargles.

So why do doctors start thinking about surgery? Most often it's because of repeated debilitating attacks of tonsillitis. There's no magic number that positively indicates tonsillectomy. But if a child is suffering from four or five severe attacks a year, it's probably time to trade antibiotics for the scalpel. Or when recurrent ear infections appear to be directly related to tonsillitis.

There's another condition called "kissing tonsils" that requires surgery. The tonsils have grown so large that they touch each other in the back of the throat. They're usually badly infected and often cause obstruction to the airway. Afflicted children become mouth-breathers, sleep poorly, tend to snore, or have long periods of apnea when they stop breathing for a minute or two.

Other children with tonsillar abscess need an operation once this severe infection subsides.

Tonsillectomy is also indicated in both adults and children when enlarged, infected tonsils are associated with halitosis. Bad breath is caused when food becomes trapped in tonsillar grooves.

Parents should realize that the majority of doctors do offer sound advice. But if a physician prescribes tonsillectomy without explanation when the child feels well, give it a second thought. Or if he suggests that other children in the family may as well have their tonsils removed at the same time, get a consultation with another doctor in a hurry. One last point. Today when surgeons are transplanting hearts and performing other miraculous procedures, no one considers that fatalities can result from simple minor operations. But on rare occasions death does occur as a result of tonsillectomy. It's a terrible tragedy when this happens. But it's a double catastrophe if the reason for the tonsillectomy was questionable in the first place.

Don't Ignore Your Child's Abdominal Pain

What is the batting average of doctors diagnosing acute appendicitis in children? Most parents would say it's high, and the diagnosis of this problem is as easy as ABC. After all, doctors have CAT scanners, x-rays, ultrasound, and other sophisticated tests these days. But to the contrary, and in spite of medical progress and modern technology, too many children are being operated on for ruptured appendix. This can have serious complications for children. So how can it be avoided?

Dr. William Clatworthy is professor of pediatric surgery at the Ohio State University. He says that nearly half of the children operated on at the Children's Hospital in Columbus, Ohio, who had a ruptured appendix had been seen earlier by a doctor who failed to suspect the problem. Some children were labeled as having a bowel upset. Others a urinary infection. Still others thought the symptoms were due to a sore throat.

Another shocking finding has emerged. One would suspect that once a child is admitted to hospital with abdominal pain a quick diagnosis would be made. But several cases of ruptured appendicitis occurred even after children were under observation in hospital.

Dr. Clatworthy's study is not an isolated finding. Dr. Harlan Stone at Grady Hospital in Atlanta reported a similar situation. Other surgeons admit that the problem is being underdiagnosed by physicians.

Why should this be the case? In the 1930s and 1940s acute appendicitis was a feared diagnosis. Parents at that time were constantly reminded that appendicitis was the seventh most common cause of death in North America. If a child suddenly complained of abdominal pain he or she was usually rushed to the doctor's office or hospital.

Doctors in the past also had a higher index of suspicion when abdominal pain struck. They knew that a missed diagnosis might mean death. So in pre-antibiotic days, only about 25 percent of cases went to the stage of perforation. But since that time, Dr. Clatworthy says, there has been a steady increase in the number of perforated appendices.

Fortunately children today have less chance of dying from a perforated appendix. But even antibiotics cannot guarantee freedom from the complications of this disease. A ruptured appendix sends large numbers of bacteria into the peritoneal cavity. In some cases of peritonitis the acute inflammatory reaction gradually subsides with little or no after-effects. But in the process of healing, scar tissue and adhesions may form that cause intestinal obstruction either months or years later. In female children the intense inflammatory reaction can cause severe damage to the fallopian tubes. If the tubes are left totally blocked, sterility results. But if only partial blockage occurs, the fertilized egg may become struck in the injured tube, causing a tubal pregnancy.

Why do today's doctors have such a poor batting average in diagnosing appendicitis? First of all it's never been an easy diagnosis in all cases. The pain may remain mild and never move to the right lower quadrant of the abdomen. In other instances, tenderness is minimal when the doctor presses on the abdomen, or he may mistake a tender, rigid abdomen as being due to the child's fear of the examination.

Deceptive symptoms abound. The presence of diarrhea or painful urination may focus the doctor's attention elsewhere. He may find little or no change in the patient's temperature or white blood cell count. Even after the appendix has ruptured and formed an abscess, the mass is passed off as due to constipation in 20 percent of cases.

Dr. Clatworthy's study revealed another interesting finding. One would think that the majority of children with an acute appendix would be examined by a surgeon. But most were seen only by the family doctor, pediatrician, or other doctors. One case in four was sent for a surgical consultation.

Why should there be so much hesitation in calling for a surgeon? Several reasons were found. There is a general reluctance for the family doctor to ask for a surgical consultation if he doesn't think the child needs an operation. He also knows that about 15 percent of children who have an operation for suspected appendicitis don't have this trouble. In recent years hospital tissue committees have come down hard on doctors who are associated with too many needless appendectomies. It's made some surgeons gun-shy about picking up the scalpel.

Parents can't improve the diagnostic skill of doctors when treating suspected acute appendicitis. But they can get their child to a doctor sooner when abdominal pain strikes. In one research study of 54 ruptured appendices, parents could be blamed in 29 of the cases for not bringing the child to the hospital soon enough.

Hemorrhoids

Hemorrhoids, like old soldiers, never die. Neither, it seems, do old medical columns. A few years ago I wrote about a new, revolutionary way to treat hemorrhoids. I still receive letters requesting information about this procedure. Is the technique just a passing gimmick? Or is the rubber band–cryosurgery operation still a proven method of treatment for this common disorder?

The technique is based on common horse sense rather than extensive sophisticated medical technology. Surgeons merely slip a rubber band over the neck of an engorged hemorrhoid. This cuts off the blood supply to the pile and it drops off in a few days. Some doctors add cryosurgery to the procedure. They use the rubber band initially; then the pile is frozen into a solid mass. Intense freezing kills the tissue, and about five days later the hemorrhoid dissolves.

There are several advantages to cryosurgery. It can be performed in a doctor's office with minimal discomfort and without the need for anesthesia. Normally a patient can return to work the same day.

There's another benefit. During a hemorrhoidectomy, the routine surgical operation for this problem, doctors occasionally remove too much tissue. This results in rectal stricture. Patients then notice that they no longer have large bowel movements. Instead they must strain to pass a stool through a smaller opening. This surgical complication can be serious. I've yet to hear of it happening with cryosurgery and the rubber band technique.

As with all surgical operations, however, there are also disadvantages to this new relatively simple method. It's usually not possible to remove all hemorrhoids in one visit. Most patients require two or three. Anyone who contemplates undergoing the procedure must realize another important fact. Even minor procedures, on rare occasions, can have frightening complications. This technique is no exception.

I knew a doctor who decided on cryosurgery for himself. Following the event he was delighted by his good fortune. God was in heaven and birds were singing. Then one day he began to feel weak. He noticed heavy rectal bleeding. On the way to the hospital he collapsed in the parking lot. Examination revealed that one of the healing hemorrhoids had started to bleed profusely. He required emergency surgery to save his life. Fortunately it's a very rare complication, and the same thing can happen when hemorrhoids are treated by surgery.

If this revolutionary method is so superior, why isn't it used by all surgeons? Some doctors argue the older technique provides good results, so why change? This is the typical conservative reaction to new methods. Only time and continued success convince some people.

But cryosurgery and the rubber band technique can no longer be classified as a passing fad. A specialist in the field, the Rudd Clinic in Toronto, reveals that it never treats hemorrhoids any other way and that the great majority of surgeons haven't taken the time to get a first-hand look at this technique. Consequently only a few North American doctors are utilizing the method.

A friend recently asked, "What would you do if you had troublesome hemorrhoids?" There's no doubt I'd select cryosurgery. I've seen it done on several occasions at the Rudd Clinic in Toronto. I've talked with post-operative patients. Everything I've seen and heard makes sense.

Do some patients require surgery to cure hemorrhoids? Dr. William Rudd, one of the pioneers of the rubber band cryosurgical technique, says some people do need a rectal "facelift." Internal hemorrhoids are always amenable to cryosurgery. But sometimes skin tags form around the rectum and become swollen. Recurrent blood clots in the same area may pose another problem. Then a combination of cryosurgery and a rectal facelift may be necessary.

Most people cringe when hemorrhoidectomy is mentioned. They therefore delay seeing a doctor when rectal bleeding occurs. They assume the bleeding is due to piles and envision days of excruciating pain after an operation. This can be a fatal error if bleeding is due to cancer. Widespread use of cryosurgery for hemorrhoids would change the public image of this disease. And people would be less apt to ignore rectal bleeding, thus curing more large bowel malignancies.

One final point. Surgeons might remember the stormy economic times upon us. They could help decrease the cost of medical care by treating most hemorrhoids in the office. This would leave costly hospital beds available for other patients. An aging population means more of us will develop this common malady. Old soldiers and hemorrhoids will never die.

Rectal Cancer and Colostomy

Thirty thousand Canadians will be struck by a double-barreled shock this year. First, a doctor will inform them they have a cancer of the rectum. Then, before they've recovered from this initial impact, the next blow will fall. They'll discover that surgery means an artificial bowel opening in the abdomen—a colostomy. It strikes terror in the hearts of most patients as they consider life with this heavy burden.

Rectal cancers occur in the last 6 inches of the large bowel. Like other malignancies, they can be present for many months without causing symptoms. But eventually one or more problems occur. Some patients notice blood in a bowel movement. Others, a change in bowel habits. This may be constipation, diarrhea, or intermittent episodes of alternating constipation with loose bowel movements. Crampy pain is normally a late symptom. And occasionally patients will become weak due to anemia from chronic blood loss.

The great majority of people with these symptoms do not have cancer. Most cases of rectal bleeding are from hemorrhoids. Similarly, constipation is often the result of faulty eating and bowel habits. But if these symptoms suddenly appear, consult a doctor immediately. The early detection of a rectal malignancy is one of the prime ways to prevent colostomy.

Luckily, new techniques are spotting early rectal and large bowel cancers. Dr. Victor Gilbertson of Minneapolis said recently, "For the price of a good bottle of whiskey you can make sure you don't die from cancer of the rectum."

He was referring to the fiberoptic colonoscope, a flexible instrument which enables surgeons to examine the rectum and the entire large bowel.

This represents a vast improvement over older methods of diagnosis. For instance, half the cancers of the large bowel occur in the rectum. The majority of these can be felt by the doctor's fingers during examination. Then, to evaluate the extent of the tumor and to detect cancers further away from the anus, the rigid sigmoidoscope was available. But this cannot get around corners to explore all the large bowel.

Now the large bowel's "outer space" has been penetrated by the colonoscope. Its use is confirming a longstanding debate about whether benign fleshy growths in the bowel, called polyps, become malignant. Dr. Gilbertson has followed 20,000 patients for seven years. His findings indicate that removal of benign polyps will prevent many future cancers.

So far there isn't a routine test like the Pap test to seek out early bowel cancers. But select population groups have been screened by another method. A small piece of the patient's stool is tested to find "occult" or hidden blood. Roughly 2 to 5 percent of those screened will have a positive result. Studies are then carried out to determine whether the presence of minute amounts of blood is due to cancer or some benign condition such as hemorrhoids.

Some surgeons I talked to in Canada and the U.S. believe the colonoscope will eliminate cancer of the rectum in this generation. I hope so. But I think the sudden disappearance of this common malignancy is an unrealistic dream. This means that thousands face the prospect of a permanent colostomy. For some, the size and location of the tumor will leave patients and surgeons no choice. But others will end their days with an unnecessary permanent colostomy. It's a tragedy when it could have been avoided.

In researching my weekly column I often encounter incredible surprises. It happened again while I was digging for the facts of rectal cancer. One would suspect that patients have enough psychological stress to contend with on learning of this diagnosis without added pressures. But I encountered unbelievable stories of conflict between medical personnel while treating patients with cancer of the rectum.

Prominent colon and rectal surgeons were hesitant to talk unless I assured anonymity. Nurses specially trained to care for colostomies were also fearful to express opinions. But piece by piece a picture took shape. Some startling and disturbing facts emerged.

An outstanding Toronto surgeon said, "I strongly agree with you that many needless colostomies are done. But preserving rectal function can be a difficult operation for inexperienced surgeons."

Another surgeon in western Canada remarked, "Doctors who don't treat much rectal cancer are unable to perform the new techniques to preserve the rectum. If the average surgeon attempted these pull-through operations the patient would end up with horrendous complications."

A U.S. rectal surgeon with impeccable credentials stated, "Some patients have radical surgery for small malignancies that could be treated by radiation or electrocoagulation. But you must know what you're doing. Patients in smaller centres can't receive the same level of care as those people treated in university hospitals. There's no doubt that needless colostomies are done by surgeons unfamiliar and inexperienced in the new procedures."

Nursing enterostomal therapists (there are 83 in Canada) made some distressing comments. It's their job to help patients adjust psychologically to a colostomy and to teach them how to care for it. The majority of surgeons welcome their help. But several remarked, "Some surgeons are terribly arrogant. They won't let us see the patient before the operation, or suggest individual locations for the colostomy. Often they select an area forgetting it's in a crease or flabby spot when the patient stands up. Being off just half an inch can make it hard to fit the colostomy bag. At other times the colostomy is too close to the belt line or too high so a young person can't wear jeans."

What does this mean for patients who develop rectal cancer? I've often said that it's the doctor who primarily determines whether patients receive top-drawer or mediocre care. Few better examples exist than patients who have surgical treatment for cancer of the rectum.

But finding skilled hands is easier said than done for the person on the street. It's a tough assignment even when you're thinking straight, and patients with rectal cancer are under great psychological stress. It means that 99 percent of the time people have little or no choice in this matter. If the cancer is close to the rectal opening, a colostomy will be automatic unless they're very lucky.

But more than luck should be at play. Chance has no role in the treatment of cervical malignancy (cancer of the lower part of the uterus) in women. Such cases are always referred to university centers for specialized care.

People deserve the same approach for low-lying rectal cancers. Family doctors should have access to the names of those who perform these new operations. The Cancer Society and Ostomy Associations should also exert pressure for more open information. Everyone agrees that early diagnosis is invaluable. But getting the best surgical care is also important.

Some surgeons believe that the colostomy operation offers the best hope of cure. But a report in the *New England Journal of Medicine* hardly justifies this opinion. The five-year survival rate after a colostomy was 50 percent. It increased to 64 percent when rectal function was preserved. Moreover, in one series, normal bowel function was maintained in 100 consecutive cases.

Several surgeons stressed that a colostomy was not a disaster. One said, "I'd rather have a colostomy than lose two of my fingers." I'd agree that many patients function well with a colostomy. But others find the adjustment difficult. They would have preferred a choice if the size and location of the malignancy had not demanded a colostomy, particularly when some of them have lost jobs because of this operation or cannot get into nursing homes because of it.

A recent U.S. book will slow the trend of needless colostomies. It's titled, *The Best Doctors in the U.S.* The author, John Pekkanen, obtained the names of 2,500 doctors by asking leading physicians, "Who would you consult for this medical problem?" It's unfortunate there isn't a Canadian edition. In the meantime, patients facing surgery for rectal malignancy should ask their doctors if they know a surgeon with experience in these new techniques.

The Urinary Bladder Can Be Saved When Cancer Strikes

What should you do if faced with this terrible news? The specialist states that the urinary bladder must be totally removed by surgery because of cancer. Should you quickly agree to the operation? Or is there a way to avoid the unpleasant prospect of wearing a bag to collect urine?

The patient is passing bloody urine. A cystoscopic examination reveals extensive malignancy. The patient is given just one choice. Nothing short of completely removing the bladder holds any hope of cure. The family, in a state of shock, agrees to proceed with the operation as advised.

But after the terror of the initial blow recedes, they fortunately have the presence of mind to seek another opinion at a university medical center. In view of the radical nature of the operation, it is decided that if the cancer is extensive, a short delay will not affect the outcome.

The second specialist offers different advice. To be sure, the bladder contains several malignant growths. But it's possible to remove them with a new technique, the insertion of a small cutting instrument into the bladder through the penis. The patient will be discharged five days after surgery, with his bladder intact and a good chance of cure. Seeking another opinion will save him from a catastrophic outcome. But how can two specialists reach diametrically opposite opinions?

I've often stressed that surgeons differ markedly in surgical skill. It's not easy to remove a large number of malignant growths from the inside of the bladder when working with a small lighted instrument. But one of these urologists has the technical skill and extensive experience to do it. The other either firmly believes that the lesser operation is the wrong way to treat the malignancy or doesn't possess the necessary skill to perform it. In any case the patient is not offered any alternative by the first consultant.

Medical consumers should keep several points in mind when faced with a problem of this magnitude. It's been aptly said that war is far too important to be left entirely to generals. Radical surgery such as total removal of a bladder is similarly too drastic to be left in the hands of one consulting physician—one who perhaps has not kept pace with the times, or whose philosophical approach refuses to accept that lesser forms of treatment are sometimes advisable. Or who refuses to refer to another surgeon who is capable of saving an organ as vital as a urinary bladder.

It's also reasonable to speculate whether this patient was fully informed at the original consultation of the consequences of radical surgery. That he had at least a 5 percent chance of not surviving the operation. That he would be left impotent. That there are often chronic complications from wearing a bag to collect urine. That his quality of life would never be the same again. Patients can learn to live reasonably well with a bowel colostomy, but with bladder removal the flow of urine never stops.

Has this man taken too much risk in agreeing to a lesser operation? I don't think so. The bladder can be checked again in a few months. If a growth is too small to be detected at the initial operation it can be removed at this time. Undergoing a cystoscopic examination at regular intervals is a small price to pay for keeping the bladder functioning.

How many needless radical operations are done in this country every year is impossible to calculate. But I'm sure that many people have colostomies of the bowel or urinary bladders removed which could have been avoided.

A professor of surgery recently commented, "We have many patients who are referred to the university for pre-operative radiation in preparation for bowel colostomy. But when we examine them we often discover it's technically feasible to remove the cancerous bowel and leave the rectum intact. We try to inform the referring surgeon as discreetly as possible that this can be done." But he had no idea how often the referring surgeon took this advice.

Be sure to consult a doctor quickly when you discover bloody urine. It might be due to a benign polyp, a urinary infection, or a kidney stone. But if it's due to bladder cancer, get another opinion if total removal of the bladder is recommended. If a university center or a major clinic is nearby, seek its advice. If there isn't, buy a plane ticket. It could save your bladder.

Surgery for Gallstones?

What would I do if a colleague told me I had gallstones? Would I agree to immediate removal of the gallbladder? Would I try to dissolve the stones with new drugs? Or would I hope the crematorium fire would eventually take care of them? It's an important question for the 16 million North Americans who have gallstones.

Several studies indicate it's wiser to leave gallstones alone. Dr. Murray M. Fisher is an Associate Professor of Medicine at the University of Toronto. In 1978 he delivered a paper, "Perspectives on Gallstones," to the International Symposium on Gallstones. He stated, "It is quite possible that 80 percent or more of subjects with gallstones can live with them and not require surgical intervention."

Other studies confirm this suspicion. Four hundred and seventy-eight Danish patients with gallstones were followed from 5 to 20 years. During that time only one quarter required surgery. Another study reported in the October 1981 *Lancet* medical journal showed that only 16 of 123 gallstone patients developed complications during a 10- to 15-year period.

Today gallstones are about as common as hens' eggs. In 1974 Swedish doctors stressed this fact in the *Scandinavian Journal of Gastroenterology*. They carried out post-mortem studies of 85 percent of the residents of Prague and of Malmo who died during the years 1963 to 1966. They found that the frequency of gallstone disease in this population was 30 percent for males and 50 percent for females. U.S. researchers found the same incidence of gallstones in the Pima and Micmac Indians.

It means that the majority of people with this disease have "silent stones." They float freely inside the gallbladder for years without causing symptoms. And many people die without ever knowing they were present.

These are better odds than at the racetrack. So why rush into surgery when someone may cremate my gallstones? Besides there's always a small risk to surgery. *The Lancet* journal states that 4 in 1,000 patients die from the operation. And 7 in 100 patients develop post-operative complications. I have no doubt that I'd keep my gallstones if they were spotted during x-ray examination for a sore back.

Would anything sway me towards surgery? Silent stones don't always remain quiescent. A small stone might be pushed out of the gallbladder. It might get trapped in the cystic duct, causing obstruction of the flow of bile and precipitate an attack of acute cholecystitis. Or the stone might progress further into the common bile duct and produce jaundice.

I'd have to experience only one acute attack of cholecystitis to agree quickly to surgery. It's much easier to remove the gallbladder between attacks than when it's badly inflamed.

Suppose I was spared an acute episode, but suffered from intermittent bouts of mild upper abdominal discomfort, bloating, and indigestion? I'd know these symptoms might be due to chronic infection in the gallbladder or the stones. But patients without stones can also have these troubles. Moreover, when the gallbladder is removed some patients are left with these same symptoms. I'd first improve my dietary lifestyle. And resort to the operation only if the symptoms became more pronounced.

Can gallstones be dissolved without surgery? In 1902 scientists isolated a substance from the bile of polar bears that spurred this hope. As a result drugs are now available that help some patients avoid an operation.

How effective is the treatment? Unfortunately neither chenodeoxycholic (CDC) or ursdeoxycholic (UDC) are the panacea for many patients. Dr. Murray Fisher emphasized that out of 100 gallstone patients only 25 are suitable for therapy.

The other 75 must bypass the drugs for several reasons. For instance, if x-rays reveal calcified cholesterol stones, there's no hope they'll dissolve. Obese patients also respond poorly to treatment. And large single stones are rarely affected, possibly due to the large surface area. Doctors are also unable to use these drugs during a woman's reproductive years.

It's not a bed of roses for the 25 percent who can take the drugs. Some patients develop indigestion and nausea. The treatment requires two years or longer. Sometimes the stones reappear once the drugs are stopped. Just 20 to 30 percent of these patients get good results.

My choice would be a first-class surgeon to remove troublesome gallstones.

But if fate presents me with silent stones, I'll run from the scalpel. I'd hope that the crematorium fire would dissolve them when I'm 90.

"Video-Game Surgery" of the Knee

Who will forget those moments of the 1984 Olympic Games? The memorable entrance of Joan Benoit into the Los Angeles stadium to win the first women's Olympic marathon race. Or the petite Mary Lou Retton winning the gold medal in gymnastics. Millions of TV watchers also learned that both medalists had undergone recent arthroscopic surgery on their knees. Since then readers have asked for information on this procedure. My mail indicates that considerable confusion exists about the nature and benefits of this operation.

The arthroscope is much like the periscope in a submarine. It's a fiberoptic viewing instrument that can be inserted into the knee for a direct look at the joint. During the past 10 years arthroscopes have been widely used in the diagnosis of joint problems that have not been detected by either physical examination or x-rays. In addition, surgeons can perform corrective surgery through this instrument.

Arthroscopic surgery is performed by inserting the arthroscope about 6 millimeters into the knee joint. A TV camera can be attached to the arthroscope and the resulting image from inside the knee projected onto a TV screen. Other instruments, usually two, are then inserted through "mini" holes to carry out the operation. Due to the complex and precise eye-hand maneuvers required, the procedure has been dubbed "video-game surgery."

The most common operation carried out by an arthroscope is a meniscectomy which removes knee cartilage. The bones of the knee joint are normally cushioned by two half-moon shaped pieces of cartilage. These cushions, located around the rim of the joint, are easily injured by the stress of a variety of athletic activities.

Dr. James Nicholas, Director of Lennox Hill Institute of Sports Medicine in New York, says the knee is the body's most vulnerable joint, the one least suited to perform what it is asked to do. That's why about 200,000 North Americans every year require either partial or complete removal of one or both damaged cartilages.

Like Joan Benoit and Mary Lou Retton, patients have to make a decision when a meniscus is damaged. One choice is to live with pain, especially during activity. And to accept the fact that occasional episodes will occur when the knee will lock because torn or loose pieces of cartilage have become jammed between the bones of the knee joint. It's not a life-threatening situation, and each person has to decide when the pain and annoyance are sufficient to proceed with surgery.

How does the removal of damaged cartilage affect the knee? Obviously the joint becomes less functional than one that has an intact meniscus. But when a patient can still win an Olympic gold medal after this surgery, it shows that adequate functioning of the knee is retained.

Another point must be considered when deciding the pros and cons of this surgery. A damaged meniscus which locks and causes pain will slowly but surely continue to injure the joint over the years. The end result is often premature degenerative joint disease. In essence, better to have half a good meniscus than retain one that is diseased.

Arthroscopic knee surgery offers several advantages over the traditional 4- to 6-inch incision. Rather than spend several days in hospital, patients usually leave the hospital hours after the operation. And instead of weeks of recuperation, walking can be resumed within 24 hours.

So why isn't all knee meniscus surgery done this way? Some forms of cartilage surgery cannot be done easily through the arthroscope. But the experts in this technique now insist that practically any type of knee cartilage surgery can and should be performed this way. The limiting factor is that few surgeons are expert enough to feel comfortable in recommending it.

What should medical consumers do when they're told the trouble is an injured meniscus requiring removal? My advice is to do what the doctors do. I don't think there are many physicians in this country today who would agree to a traditional incision to excise knee cartilage. They know that the only way to go to surgery is on a first-class ticket. They would find a surgeon who has removed hundreds of damaged cartilages using the arthroscope. Ask your doctor to refer you to one of these surgeons. There's no doubt that video-game surgery is here to stay.

The Facelift: Slightly More than a New Hairstyle.

Betty Ford, wife of a former U.S. President, has a new face. She explained, "I'm 60 years old and wanted a nice new face to go with my beautiful new life." Her action is symptomatic of a new boom in cosmetic surgery, and her public announcement will feed the fire. But women should tread lightly before they rush into this latest fad. Before-and-after photographs don't tell the whole story. Choosing a new face is not quite as easy as changing the hairstyle.

The facelift is not minor surgery. Don't be misled into thinking that the plastic surgeon makes a few quick pleats and tucks and produces a brand-new, unblemished appearance. Extensive incisions are often required. And as in any surgical procedure, potential trouble always lurks in the operating room.

Consider a recent report on 922 facelifts. The average age of the patients was 54, but amazingly some were in their late 20s and early 30s. There were 181 major complications. The biggest problem was sloughing of the skin. Some patients developed large blood clots under the skin flaps. Others were left with unsightly scars that required further surgery. And six had weakness of the facial muscle due to injury of the facial nerve.

Remember that plastic surgeons, although highly skilled, are not demi-gods. They can't make you look like Sophia Loren or Robert Redford. Some people enter surgery with such false hopes. And often the surgeon's concept of a satisfactory result is quite different from the expectation of the patient.

Even plastic surgery of the nose is fraught with risk. One young woman, tired of being teased about her Bob Hope nose, chose a straightening procedure. Her surgeon thought he achieved a superb result. But the patient, proud of her Irish identity, was not expecting to lose all the curve of her profile. She cried hysterically when she saw her new straight "Roman" nose.

Plastic surgery of the face is not like shopping at Eaton's. Some new faces are devastatingly unexpected, or changed for the worse. But you can't return them to the exchange department in return for the old one.

Another drawback of facelifts is rarely mentioned. They last only four to eight years. There are no reports to evaluate the psychological effect on patients as the new face also begins to wrinkle or sag. Do you consider another facelift? Does it trigger severe depression? Or do you finally accept the aging process gracefully?

Trick photography also plays a part in the before-and-after pictures. Betty Ford's recent photos reveal a new softer hairdo. Her dress has a lower neckline or a soft scarf. A wider smile shows sparkling white teeth. Perhaps new make-up completes the effect. One make-up expert says, "It's a matter of giving a woman glorious cheeks." Plastic surgery textbooks use the same tricks in their before-and-after photos.

Bear in mind, too, that cosmetic surgery of the face does not rejuvenate the body. It can't provide new arteries, a better digestive system, or improved physical wellbeing. It might mean tauter skin on the top with varicose veins on the bottom. Nor can it erase emotional insecurities. The workings that go on inside the skull remain the same, and may even be burdened with yet another major adjustment. Remember, what we are inside can't be changed by the plastic surgeon's scalpel.

Then there is the consideration of expense. A 50-year-old woman writes from the Maritimes that she visited a plastic surgeon in one of our major cities. Although not unattractive, she was offered a new improved appearance at a cost of $4,000.

When compared with other surgery, often more hazardous, this is extravagant. The removal of cancerous organs, transplanting of kidneys and repairing of damaged hearts, is more threatening. Yet these surgeons measure their fees in hundreds of dollars.

No doubt there are men and women who have successful results from cosmetic surgery. Perhaps they are happier for a time. But it would be interesting to study their reactions after 5 or 10 years. Would it be worth it? I suspect there would be those who said no.

We have not yet found the way to delay the aging process. It is relentless. No amount of glamorous trappings or trick photography can slow it. Nor will smooth skin help us accept it any better.

9

Is There an Ideal Contraceptive?

Some days I'm astounded at the needless medical problems I see: A 45-year-old mother of three who expects to be a grandmother, but finds herself pregnant; an 18-year-old girl, scheduled to start college, who must accept motherhood instead; the 23-year-old secretary who wanted simply to postpone pregnancy, but now faces life without children. These catastrophes happen when women use the wrong contraceptive at the wrong time. But such tragedies can be avoided.

Never believe that the perfect contraceptive exists for everyone. Some women have little choice in the method of birth control they select. For others it's vital to choose the contraceptive that suits the personality.

Some young girls have no option. A married student who wishes to complete a college degree requires a 100 percent contraceptive. The birth control pill is the only one that fits this category. This young woman should forget about the one in a million chance of pill complications if she enjoys good health. The risk of unwanted pregnancy far outweighs the tales one hears about the dangers of the pill. In actual fact it has an enviable safety record. We all face greater dangers every day.

Young girls also frequently entertain the wrong idea about the IUD. They believe naively that they can insert the intra-uterine device easily and all will be well. But the device can be very difficult, if not impossible, to insert in the office in some women who haven't had a child. It can also instigate serious pelvic infection. I'll never forget one young woman who consulted me during her honeymoon. She had a huge pelvic abscess and spent the next month in hospital. Most likely she faces a life without children because of tubal injury from an IUD. This device should be used later in life.

Some couples require only 96 percent protection. They would prefer postponing pregnancy for a few years, but it wouldn't be a major disaster if pregnancy occurred earlier. These women should consider a vaginal contraceptive cream as a safe and effective interim means of birth control.

What about the woman who has completed her family and needs birth control for the remaining years of fertility? Here's where trouble awaits if the contraceptive doesn't fit the personality. Both patient and doctor should consider some critical questions before making a decision.

What would happen if contraception failed? Would religious or moral principles allow the patient to submit to an abortion? Are abortions readily available in that part of the country? Or would it mean an unwanted pregnancy at 40?

Women who can accept abortion may decide on a vaginal contraceptive cream. These creams are highly effective, but they must be used conscientiously; they can't be used one night, then left in the drawer the next. Patients who are apt to play Russian roulette with creams should have an IUD inserted. A few will be bothered by troublesome bleeding. Others will expel the device. But the majority will tolerate it without problems for many years.

If abortion is unthinkable a 96 percent contraceptive won't do. Then two choices are open: continuing to take the birth control pill or sterilization.

Can the pill be used for a prolonged period of time? This is a reasonable alternative in some cases. Some women feel great while taking the pill. Others enjoy the feeling of security it provides. Giving up the pill causes too much worry. So why substitute a stomach ulcer or hypertension?

There are qualifying conditions if the pill is to be selected for the final reproductive years. It will be safer if the patient does not smoke and is not overweight. Also the Pap smear must remain normal. There shouldn't be a history of diabetes in the family. Visual difficulties, increasing headaches, or pains in the legs or chest indicate an immediate need to switch to another form of birth control.

Sterilization is accepted today by an increasing number of women. The age-old method involves an incision to cut and tie off the fallopian tubes. I prefer laparoscopy. A periscope-like instrument is inserted into the abdomen through a half-inch cut just below the navel. It enables the surgeon to either cauterize the tubes or place plastic clamps on them. Laparoscopy is performed in hospital, but is less painful than the traditional tubal ligation, and most patients return home the same day.

I'd be able to stop shaking my head in astonishment if patients would read a little Shakespeare. He gave sage advice in Henry VI when he wrote, "Defer no time; delays have dangerous ends." He could have been talking about teenagers and potential grandmothers who delay the decision about birth control.

The Oral Contraceptive Controversy

There has never been a pill quite like the birth control pill. It's been available for over 20 years. To the over 50 million women taking it every day, it has finally given freedom from the fear of an unwanted pregnancy. However, unlike other pills, it has continued to be surrounded by controversy, apprehension, and half-truths. Some of this alarm has been generated by scare headlines, such as, "Why 1,000,000 women stopped the pill," or, "Study links heart attacks to the pill." The medical profession has also added fuel to the fire.

I've received numerous letters asking about the pill. Mrs. E.D. of Prince

George wrote, "I'm 41 and I've been on the pill for 12 years. Is it dangerous to stay on it any longer?" Another reader from Halifax questioned, "I've been told that the pill causes cancer. I'm afraid to stay on it and terrified to stop it. Would you give me your opinion?" Other letters have asked if the pill causes diabetes or should it be taken if fibroids are present.

Why has the pill developed such a questionable reputation in some circles? Part of the reason can be answered on solid medical grounds. For instance, it's been shown that the pill tends to produce blood clots in the legs and other areas, which can result in death in about five out of every million users. It may also have an adverse effect on the menstrual period and the ability to become pregnant later on. Other studies indicate that, in susceptible patients, it may hasten the onset of high blood pressure and diabetes. There is no doubt that these women and others should think twice before going on the pill and that a few patients should never start it, but remember, before you throw your pills away, that 85 percent of women in the reproductive age can safely take the pill. Never, never forget that many of the pill's woes have resulted from moral, ethical, and religious debates rather than purely medical ones. That's why the pill has had a tougher road to travel than aspirin, penicillin, and other less controversial drugs. People die from penicillin reactions and from a variety of other drug problems, but these cases seldom hit the headlines.

There are few things in life as safe as the birth control pill. For example, for every 200,000 people, 54 die in car accidents and another 35 succumb from childbirth. Yet only about one woman has a fatal reaction to the pill. That's an extremely good track record for a drug that has received such screaming headlines, but just as some people can't eat peanuts, so should some women bypass the pill.

First of all there are a few 100 percent contraindications to the use of the pill. For instance, women who have had phlebitis, an injured liver, or a suspected cancer of the breast must not take the pill. Similarly, patients who have undiagnosed vaginal bleeding or an early pregnancy should not take it, but there are some grey areas where you can go one way or the other. The older woman who has been on the pill for 15 years is a case in question. Should she continue to take it until she is 50 years of age, or would it be wiser to switch to another means of contraception? Part of this answer must come from the doctor and part from the patient.

The 40-year-old woman can feel secure about the pill if regular check-ups continue to be normal. In short, there is no magic age when she should stop the pill, nor is there a definite limit to the number of years it can be taken, but getting older is not always free of problems whether you are on or off the pill. Some women have a tendency to show the early tell-tale symptoms of hypertension. Others become obese and the doctor may detect a small amount of sugar in the urine. These women would be advised to stop the pill since there is some evidence that it may accelerate these problems. There is no point in pushing your luck, particularly when other contraceptives are available. Yet some women may still decide to accept this small additional risk rather than switching to another less reliable contraceptive.

There are also some young women who should shy away from the pill—for instance, those who have a history of infrequent, irregular periods are poor candidates for this method of contraception. To be sure, the pill will produce regular monthly bleeding, and that's the very thing that springs the trap. The pill works by giving the pituitary and hypothalamic glands a rest. The problem is that formerly lazy glands sometimes get used to this vacation and don't want to return to work. Women who were born with a fragile hormonal system may find that it takes many months before the periods return once the pill has been stopped. Others may require the use of drugs to stimulate these glands into action. It can at times be a dicey problem for the young woman who wants to become pregnant at a later date.

Women of all ages should say no to the pill if they suffer from migraine headaches or epilepsy or if they develop severe depression after being on the pill for several months, and if women are having intercourse at very infrequent intervals it may be better to stop the pill and use other types of contraceptives.

What about cancer? For instance, is there any proof that the pill causes cancer of the breast? Fortunately after over 20 years there is still no evidence that its continued use results in this malignancy. In fact, two separate studies have shown that women on the pill are less susceptible to developing either benign tumours or cystic disease of the breast. It's worthwhile remembering that breast cancer and the other malignancies were around long before anyone had ever heard of the pill.

What should you do if your doctor tells you to avoid the pill? Go along with his advice if you've developed severe headaches, visual problems, pains in the legs or chest, or some of the other difficulties I've mentioned. Moreover if you're the type who frequently forgets to take the pill and it's causing abnormal bleeding, don't be surprised if the doctor throws up his hands and suggests something else.

Most doctors will give sound advice on the pill, but anyone can get trapped by physicians who have Ethical Pill Disease. These doctors tend to overestimate the liabilities of the pill and minimize its great assets. They seem to use every excuse in the book to steer patients away from this reliable form of contraception. Possibly their worst error is to advise a temporary holiday from the pill when there's no proven reason to stop it if you're feeling fine, tests are normal, and you've never suffered from those lazy periods. Too often a pill vacation ends with an unwanted pregnancy.

Good News About the Pill

Doubting Thomases should remember Plutarch's remark in 46 A.D., "Time is the wisest of counselors." Years of needless worry could be avoided. When the birth control pill burst on the medical scene 20 years ago it was immediately and relentlessly criticized by skeptics in both the medical and popular press. The pill became the whipping boy for a variety of political, religious, and ethical groups. A few of us maintained that time would prove that the benefits of the pill far outweighed the small risk involved in its prolonged use. Two decades later, has the birth control pill withstood the test of time?

The Royal College of General Practitioners in Great Britain conducted a major study of the pill in 1968. They compared the health of 23,611 women on the pill with 22,766 women of the same age and social class not using oral contraceptives.

Some findings were predictable. Oral contraceptive users were half as likely to develop iron deficiency anemia due to decreased menstrual flow. This benefit continued even after women stopped the pill. The increase in iron stores remained in the body for several years.

But there were some very surprising findings. Oral contraceptive users were less likely to develop cancer of the uterus, benign ovarian tumors, fibrocystic disease of the breast, and pelvic infection were less likely to need pelvic surgery. Several other studies in the U.S. since that time have confirmed these findings, but they have yet to receive their fair share of publicity.

Patients will no doubt continue to ask me if the pill causes cancer. This is a notion difficult to dispel. But now we know the reverse is true. Women on the birth control pill have a 50 percent less chance of developing cancer of the uterus. Moreover, the longer the oral contraceptives are used, the greater the protective effect. This reduced risk of uterine cancer also lasts for five years after the pills are stopped.

More than 10 published studies indicate that oral contraceptives help to safeguard the breast from cystic disease. For instance a report in *The New England Journal of Medicine* in 1976 revealed that women who took the pill for more than two years had a 65 percent reduction in fibrocystic disease of the breast. As with cancer of the uterus, there was a further decrease with longer usage.

How does the birth control pill protect against these problems? Estrogen has a stimulating effect on both the lining of the uterus and on breast tissue. It's believed that the progesterone component of the pill helps to cushion the estrogen effect.

Further good news comes from Scandinavia. A study conducted at the University Hospital in Linkoping, Sweden, revealed that oral contraceptives also provide protection against pelvic infection. Women with gonorrhea on the pill had half the chance of getting an acute infection of the fallopian tubes. Researchers postulated the increased protection was related to the decreased duration of menstrual flow. This permits fewer germs to travel through the uterus to the tubes.

Dr. Howard W. Orgy is chief of Family Planning at the Centers for Disease Control in Atlanta. He reported last year to fertility experts gathered in

Leuven, Belgium, that the preventive effects of the pill were substantial. His studies compared 100,000 women using oral contraceptives with the same number not taking the pill.

His results? For pill users there were 235 fewer cases yearly of benign breast disease, 600 fewer cases of pelvic infection, 120 fewer cases of tubal pregnancy, 35 fewer cases of ovarian cysts, and 300 fewer cases of iron deficiency anemia. Pill users also appeared to have a lower risk of developing rheumatoid arthritis. These women also had 270 fewer operations every year to remove ovarian cysts and benign cysts of the breast.

Time has obviously vindicated the birth control pill. For years it's helped to relieve women of troublesome menstrual problems and fear of an unwanted pregnancy. These other documented bonuses should go a long way to end the witch hunt that has pursued the pill since its inception.

The I.U.D.

"What a butcher! I'll never go back to him!" a patient recently complained to me about another doctor. This surgeon's error wasn't that he had removed the wrong leg, or left a sponge in the abdomen during surgery. He'd simply inserted an intra-uterine device (IUD) for birth control in the wrong patient. For some women this experience merely leaves bad memories. For others it has catastrophic results.

Teenage girls often request the insertion of an IUD. Some have never used any contraceptive before. But the majority are using the birth control pill and are apprehensive about its dangers. They believe the IUD can be easily inserted, has no side effects and their worry will be a thing of the past. They're invariably surprised when I report that the IUD is also risky. That I normally never advise it for their age group. And that if the pill isn't causing them problems they should continue it.

Why am I hesitant to use the IUD for teenagers? Or for young married women who have never had a child? There are several reasons. The insertion of an IUD into the uterus is always accompanied by the chance of infection. On rare occasions the procedure or the device can cause a major complication.

A few months ago I was called to see a 19-year-old girl in the emergency department of the hospital. She was on her honeymoon and had had an IUD inserted by her doctor two weeks before her marriage. When I examined her, she had a temperature of 104° F and a massive pelvic abscess. Her condition was acute, requiring prolonged hospitalization.

What a catastrophic way to start marriage! Worse still, this young bride may be permanently sterile as a result of the overwhelming infection, or require a hysterectomy later in life due to extensive scarring of the tubes and ovaries. Such an extreme result rarely happens. But I believe the risk is one that young girls need not assume or treat lightly, particularly when other effective contraceptives are available.

What prompted my patient to refer so vehemently to her doctor as a butcher? The reason was that she had never been pregnant, and childless women often have a small rigid opening into the uterus which is difficult and painful to dilate. Sometimes it's impossible to insert an IUD in such patients without the aid of an anesthetic. Her experience had obviously been painful and traumatic.

Pregnancy is another reason for being cautious about the IUD. Approximately 3 out of every 100 IUD users become pregnant in a year. If pregnancy is totally unacceptable, the birth control pill is a safer and better choice.

Some older women should circumvent the IUD. For instance, those who have heavy, prolonged, or frequent periods are poor candidates for the loop. In the majority of cases, placing a foreign body inside the uterus will aggravate these troubles. Similarly, women who have fibroid growths or a past history of pelvic infection should steer clear of the IUD.

Who, then, should use the IUD? There are some for whom this device is an excellent means of contraception. For women who have had multiple pregnancies, it's usually a simple matter to insert the IUD. Moreover, these patients are older, further reducing the chance of pregnancy.

The IUD is also useful in spacing pregnancies. Some women are unsure whether or not they want more children. Others may not seek pregnancy but are willing to accept it if it happens. Older women approaching menopause often want the added assurance of this device.

How does the IUD work? This foreign body, inserted inside the uterus, creates a hostile environment for the female egg. It does this by causing irritation and minor inflammation of the endometrial lining of the uterus.

The prime time for insertion is either during a period or immediately following it. The cervical opening is easier to dilate at this point and there's also less chance of pregnancy being already present. Blood loss from the procedure is also less in the early part of the menstrual cycle.

How long should an IUD be left in place? The answer to this question depends on whom you ask. Dr. Waldeman A. Schmidt, professor of gynecology at the Texas Health Sciences Center, Houston, believes it should be replaced every two years. It's been his experience that women who have an IUD in place for six years are more likely to develop pelvic infection.

He may be right. But unless an IUD is causing troublesome discharge, menstrual irregularities, pain, or fever, I normally suggest leaving it in place for several years. But remember, the initial insertion is always associated with mild discomfort and irregular bleeding. This may last for a few weeks.

My advice to women who want children eventually is that they shouldn't press their doctors into inserting an IUD. They'll thereby avoid a hazard, a possibly traumatic experience, and the feeling that their physicians were brutally sadistic!

Sterilization—A Prelude to Hysterectomy?

An operating room scrub nurse keeps prodding me to write about post-sterilization complications. Like many women she's convinced that this procedure is usually the prelude to hysterectomy, or at least initiates troublesome menstrual problems. If I delay much longer, she may soon hand me the wrong end of the scalpel.

The number of female sterilizations has skyrocketed in recent years as a result of public demand and a change in lifestyle. In the past sterilization was reserved for women with large families. Today the two-child family is considered adequate by some, mandatory by others. Some couples and career women make a firm commitment to a childless existence. But is this liberal approach causing any harm?

My scrub nurse thinks so. Some of her friends, following the operation, have developed heavy, irregular, or prolonged bleeding. Others complain of painful periods. She has suggested that I take up the scalpel again and perform hysterectomies on these patients.

In researching the facts about sterilization, I've been struck by how little textbooks have to say about it. One 1,200-page gynecology text doesn't even mention the procedure. And a recent one I was asked to review devotes just 10 lines to it. You have to dig into journals to get facts, but even they didn't provide answers on a silver platter. Researchers have a habit of disagreeing with one another.

For instance, some studies concluded that menstrual disturbances occurred in only 3 percent of cases. Others reported that abnormal bleeding and pain could be as high as 50 percent. Yet another major scrutiny of 8,500 women revealed that sterilization can also decrease the menstrual loss.

How often does sterilization lead to hysterectomy? One journal stated that 18 percent of sterilized women eventually came to this operation. But it is easy to be tricked by figures unless you read the fine print. For example, the small print brought out a rather startling fact. It said that 70 percent of women requiring hysterectomy had delivered five or more children. I'd like to remind those male authors that this in itself is no small undertaking. Would women doctors with children have reached the same conclusion? I think it's highly unlikely. They would be more tuned into how the repetitive trauma of childbirth leaves its scars on the female organs.

It's hard to pinpoint some of these post-obstetrical troubles. Some are obvious. The stretching of the vagina and supporting structures in delivery may result in the falling down of the uterus. The study showed that some of the hysterectomies were done for this reason. But female physicians wouldn't have reserved this information for the fine print.

Remember Jack Benny when you link sterilization to later problems. Everyone has a touch of this famous comedian in him. We'd all like to remain 39. And we hate to admit that our medical problems could be due to advancing age. It's much easier on the psyche to find some other scapegoat.

Remember, too, that in the past most women were sterilized in their mid to late 30s. Five years later they're 40. It's a time when fibroids, menopausal bleeding, and other gynecological disorders are more common. It's the logical sequence of the cart following the horse. A simple tying or burning of fallopian tubes probably doesn't cause these problems. Getting older does.

Don't forget that women who have been sterilized also get cancer, diabetes, strokes, and ingrown toenails. No one tries to associate these disorders with a sterilization procedure. They realize that greying hair and many other factors come into play.

There was at least some good news in the fine print. Ninety percent of women studied said they were happy the operation had been done. And many reported that the procedure had improved their sex lives.

I think my scrub nurse should accept the operation for what it is. It just blocks the tubes and leaves ovaries alone. You have to have a vivid imagination to believe this simple technique could cause serious problems.

The female consumer should be wary of a recommendation in one journal. It argued that, because of possible sterilization complications, hysterectomy should be considered a primary means of sterilization. This is currently being done more and more in the U.S. I think it's like amputating the arm when cutting off the finger would do.

Pregnancy at Fifty?

How should you look at pregnancy between 45 and 50 years of age? Can you let your guard down and still be safe from an unwanted pregnancy? Or does it require a different set of rules at this time of life? There is little doubt that most women would prefer to be a grandmother than a mother at 50. But now and then they end up changing diapers. At a time when their interests should move in other directions, they are once again trapped in child-raising. How often does it happen? Just as important, how can it be prevented?

Women of all ages are too often careless about pregnancy. You merely have to look at the vast number of abortions all over the world to grasp the immense nature of the problem. Yet even this does not tell the whole story. Many women who do not want to be pregnant nevertheless carry on with it. Some are forced to do so. Others refuse to subject themselves to an abortion.

A reckless approach to contraception is bad enough during the prime reproductive years. It is totally foolhardy in the late 40s. Yet a woman in this age group often believes that she cannot become pregnant. It's been years since she had a child, often without using any means of birth control. The periods have started to be less frequent. None of her friends are having children. And in looking at her husband it's obvious to her that he doesn't have the bounce in his step of former years. For a variety of ill-conceived reasons, she thinks it simply can't and won't happen to her.

Women's emotions tell them one thing, but hospital statistics are much more reliable. Every record room can pull out of their files the charts of patients who suddenly find themselves pregnant at this age. Fortunately nature brings on a miscarriage for some of them. Others are not so lucky.

Some women ask me, "Is it really possible to become pregnant at this age?" They seem to think that something happens to them that raises a protective wall against pregnancy. It's an emotional feeling that is partly correct—but being partly correct is where the danger lies. It's the very thing that produces those hospital statistics.

Nature does form a semi-protective screen around women at this age. Yet it also helps to confuse the game and gives a sense of false security. The ovaries, like all parts of the body, gradually age and become sluggish. Eggs are produced on a very unreliable schedule. This on-and-off ovulation now and then results in an unwanted pregnancy if women become negligent about contraception.

Is there a time when women can stop fretting about becoming an elderly mother? A good rule of thumb is that pregnancy is exceedingly unlikely once the periods have been absent for six months. And if symptoms of the menopause, such as hot flushes, are present, it's reasonable to assume that the chance of becoming pregnant is virtually nil.

What should patients do in this transitory phase when the periods may be occurring just every few months? The only way is to take the guesswork out of the game. This means using some means of contraception that is suitable for you. There isn't a good contraceptive for everyone; the choice depends on a number of factors. Women who are on the pill should consider staying on it for a few more years. Switching to another contraceptive just for the sake of switching makes no sense if the patient is doing well on this medication. The pill gives total security. Its main disadvantage is in putting a mask over the onset of the menopause. This is because all birth control pills contain estrogen, and as long as there are adequate amounts of this hormone the change of life will not begin. The only way to determine if the menopause has started is to stop the pill and see if the periods will still occur. If they do continue you should go back on the pill for another year or two. But remember to use a vaginal contraceptive while this trial period is going on. Some women don't and end up pregnant.

You can use the same approach with the coil or intra-uterine device (IUD). If it's not causing any trouble, keep it in for at least six months after the periods have stopped. Similarly, if the primary method has been either a vaginal cream or condom, these should be continued on for the same length of time.

What about the woman who hasn't used any means of contraception for years? She may suddenly become worried, think her luck has run out, and ask for advice. Is there an ideal method for her? Here you can come closer to pinpointing one, since this type of patient has no recent track record with the newer contraceptives. It is usually better to steer away from the pill at this age.

I also shy away from the IUD; abnormal bleeding is more common in the 40s, and this device may aggravate it. A vaginal cream or foam is usually the preferable method. It's effective and safe.

Is there any place for sterilization in the 40s? It's desirable in certain instances. Some women cannot tolerate the pill. Others either have irregular bleeding or expel the IUD. Still others dislike the inconvenience of a vaginal cream and live in fear that they will become pregnant. In these cases a laparoscopy sterilization should be considered.

Some patients in their early 40s who are still menstruating say the doctor assured them they couldn't become pregnant. If they heard their doctor correctly, they should not believe it unless he has valid reason for this remark. Admittedly pregnancies are less common at this time, but it is better to be careful now than sorry later.

10

Pregnancy

Don't Expect Miracles From Your Obstetrician

There's an ill wind blowing in obstetrical wards that's giving doctors a chill. Some women mistakenly believe that obstetricians have become magicians. They're convinced that every pregnancy will result in a healthy child, that there's no valid reason for any woman to die during childbirth. If it does happen, the doctor must have committed a grievous error. It's time to remind families that elaborate equipment cannot always prevent a baby's death, and the responsibility for some maternal deaths may even fall on the victim herself.

Why are doctors on the obstetrical hot seat? Like the Montreal Canadiens hockey team, they've simply been too successful. Today's obstetrical mortality rate has plunged, so people forget that just a few decades ago thousands of women and babies died in childbirth. Some mothers hemorrhaged to death. Others succumbed to fulminating infection. Or mother and child died from exhaustion after days of unproductive labor.

These problems are now past history due to antibiotics, improved prenatal care, blood transfusions, better anesthesia and surgical technique. It's made patients and families smug about childbirth. More and more the public has grown to expect the impossible from the obstetrician.

Another development is plaguing doctors. Many labor rooms now resemble a scene from *Star Wars*. During childbirth patients are surrounded by a maze of complex equipment. Machines called fetal monitors are attached to the mother and her baby. Electrodes keep track of the baby's heart rate. Others determine the frequency and strength of uterine contractions. If the baby appears to be getting into trouble, a quick caesarean section can be done.

This *Star Wars* atmosphere often makes families jump to the wrong conclusion. They reason, "How could anything happen when doctors have so much fancy apparatus monitoring the patient?" But even with all these technological advances, pregnant women and the newborn can be struck by disaster. Like the errant puck that strikes and injures a hockey player, it's the risk of the game and usually no one's fault.

Today there are new hazards for both mothers and babies. We have entered the age of what is referred to as "high risk obstetrics." And new rules must be applied to gage the success or failure of these cases. For example, in former years diabetic women often died long before reaching their reproductive years; others could not become pregnant or suffered a miscarriage due to the disease. Now, because of insulin, many can become pregnant and deliver well babies. The majority of such patients do well. But you cannot expect them to be as risk-free as others without the disorder. Similarly, women with heart and kidney disease place additional problems on the obstetrician's shoulders.

It's not only specific disease that tips the scale towards complications and sometimes maternal death. Families and newspaper headlines often neglect to mention one vital fact following obstetrical tragedies: The patient may have been her own worst enemy.

Obesity is not a cosmetic problem in obstetrics. It can be the cause of a variety of complications. Some women develop toxemia associated with hypertension, excessive swelling and urinary changes. Others will have prolonged labor and traumatic deliveries due to obstructing fat. Still others present the anesthetist with major problems, as obese patients are more difficult to anesthetize. If, for example, an obese patient arrives at the hospital in labor having just consumed a large plate of spaghetti, general anesthetic becomes more hazardous. But giving a 250-pound woman in labor a spinal or epidural anesthetic can also be technically difficult. If something goes wrong, threatening fingers invariably point at the doctors. They should be taking aim at the fat.

Luckily, doctors can forestall many obstetrical problems. But they have no sleight-of-hand tricks to prevent all troubles. The after-birth may suddenly separate prematurely from the uterus, causing severe fetal distress and death to the baby before caesarean section can be done. The complications happen under the best of conditions with the most skilled specialist. No one is to blame. There are times when even Wayne Gretzky can't put the puck in the net.

It is illogical to assume that the wheel of chance no longer spins in obstetrics as in other areas of medicine. A massive amount of electronic equipment won't put an end to the hazards of childbirth. And never forget that a patient's lifestyle, the condition of her own body and mind, can often be the determining factor in some of these tragedies.

Just Mad Dogs and Englishmen Go Out in the Noonday Sun?

When Noel Coward penned these famous words, there were no pregnant joggers in the world. Today many pregnant women continue an exercise program during pregnancy. But is strenuous exercise safe for the baby? Or is it wiser to take a quiet stroll in the garden?

Women have various reasons for exercising during pregnancy. Some use activity to control weight and appearance. Others find it relieves tension or helps prepare them for an easier labor. But what does exercise do to mother and baby?

Dr. G.J. Erdelyi carried out a study on 172 pregnant athletes. Sixty-six percent continued usual sports activities for the first three to four months. He found that their labor was only half as long as non-athletes. They had the same number of miscarriages, half the rate of caesarean sections, and fewer cases of toxemia of pregnancy.

Dr. E. Dale and other researchers showed that the heart rate of pregnant long-distance runners decreased from 125 to 140 beats per minute to 90 to 115 beats a minute. They concluded that this slowing of the mother's heart rate might be a cause for concern.

In 1978 Dr. L.D. Longo reported what happened to pregnant sheep when they exercised on a treadmill for 45 minutes. He found the fetal oxygen level decreased 19 percent. But blood flow to the uterus had a dramatic drop of 60 percent. The sheep also delivered smaller lambs. It's risky, however, to conclude that what happens in sheep also occurs in humans.

There's another potential pitfall. Comparing humans with other humans is also questionable. Most medical research of exercise during pregnancy has been done on trained athletes. Pregnant women who try to emulate their well-conditioned peers seen in sports magazines could be headed for trouble.

The advice pregnant women receive also depends on their doctor's attitude towards sports during pregnancy. Dr. James Metcalfe, a professor at the University of Oregon, says, "Studies show that in healthy women, moderate exercise doesn't seem to harm the baby. But I have no interest in advising exhaustive exercise." Metcalfe continues, "I don't think strenuous exercise is common sense. Some women may get away with it, just as some people may get away with driving drunk, but I wouldn't recommend it."

Dr. Jack Ballard, a specialist in sports medicine in Calgary, says, "there's a lot of ignorance" among physicians about exercise during pregnancy because there has been little research in this area. He worries about what happens to body temperature and the oxygen supply to the fetus.

For example, Dr. Donald McNellis at the National Institute of Child Health says, "Mothers should monitor their temperature during jogging and limit its rise to $1\frac{1}{2}$ to 2 degrees Fahrenheit."

Dr. Rudolph, a specialist in cardiovascular diseases at the William Beaumont Hospital in Royal Oak, Michigan, says a pregnant woman can exercise 20 to 40 minutes every other day at an intensity less than 85 percent of her maximum heart rate.

But some physicians gave advice that would make the late flying ace, Baron von Richthofen, rollover in his grave. For instance one doctor says that a woman's physical stability should determine her capability of participating in alpine and Nordic skiing. Other doctors agreed that activities such as gymnastics, horseback riding, hockey, and basketball carry the risk of injury by collision and the impossibility of predicting an opponent's actions; that although swimming is suitable it's wise to keep away from scuba diving; and that if a woman is very competitive in tennis, her temperature may reach a dangerous level for the fetus.

What is my advice? I wouldn't blame Baron von Richthofen for rolling over in his grave. After all how can a pregnant female skier's stability ever be guaranteed on an alpine slope? Even the best unencumbered skiers fall now and then. But what would happen if you strapped a watermelon to the waist of Jean-Claude Killy? Women who insist on skiing during pregnancy should first consult a psychiatrist. The pleasure simply isn't worth the risk.

If pregnant women want to jog on a hot summer's day, they automatically join the ranks of mad dogs and Englishmen. Common sense tells us that body temperature will rise and a decrease in oxygen supply to the fetus will occur. Currently we do not know the exact degree of oxygen deprivation. But if we are concerned with a lack of oxygen in women who smoke, we should be equally concerned with this potential problem during strenuous exercise. I'm sure Noel Coward would agree.

Career Women and the "Mañana Pregnancy"

Mrs. S.D. of Vancouver writes, "I'm 28, happily married and love my work. Eventually we want a family, but I would like to delay it as long as possible. How safe is it to have a child in your 30s? Would I require a caesarean section?"

Another reader, Ms. C.P. of Ottawa asks, "I'm a 100 percent career woman with no desire to marry or have a child. But if I have a change of heart later in life what troubles might I run into? Is there much chance of an abnormal child?"

More and more, North American women are planning for a mañana baby. Some women are finding new and exciting challenge in business. Others prefer a childless marriage for several years. Still other couples are unable to decide whether or not they ever want children.

Women whose lifestyles are so predicated should be aware of some potential pitfalls. Putting off things until tomorrow can be hazardous in many situations, and pregnancy is no exception.

For one thing a mañana baby may never appear. Today it's easy to forget this basic fact. After all, everyone reads that hundreds of thousands of needless abortions are done every year in Canada and the U.S. It's also common knowledge that millions of women are preventing pregnancy by the birth control pill. On the surface it would appear that avoiding an unwanted child is the main problem.

Career women should not make the mistake of thinking that pregnancy at any age is as simple as flicking on a light switch. Remember that one couple in 10 is infertile for a variety of reasons. Delaying a pregnancy till the middle years lowers the batting average.

Failure to have a manana baby can result from a number of problems. Some women are born with a weak menstrual system which causes infrequent and irregular periods in early life, usually because feeble ovaries fail to ovulate at monthly intervals. If lazy ovaries have trouble producing eggs in the 20s, it's easy to predict they'll have more difficulty doing so in the 30s.

Pelvic disease may also enter the picture. Some women in their 30s will develop fibroids, ovarian cysts, endometriosis, or pelvic infection, which will decrease the possibility of pregnancy.

Who knows what the future will bring? I recall one patient who was always postponing pregnancy when she suddenly developed acute appendicitis during a vacation in Europe. It ruptured prior to surgery and ended her chances of pregnancy by severely blocking both fallopian tubes.

Women who eventually have a mañana pregnancy face other potential problems. More of these patients will have a miscarriage, toxemia of pregnancy, difficult labor, or late pregnancy bleeding that requires a caesarean section. Doctors have to handle these women with kid gloves during the entire nine months.

Mañana pregnancies are also more likely to produce abnormal babies. For instance, between the ages of 35 and 39, one in 280 births are mongoloid. Between 40 and 44, one in 70, and between 45 and 49, one in 40.

If you're planning a mañana pregnancy, see your doctor every year so that he has a chance of spotting early troubles that might change your long-term planning. A Pap smear may begin to show minimal abnormal changes. A small fibroid might start to increase in size. Or the doctor may detect the internal bleeding associated with endometriosis that could scar the female organs.

The best advice is not to push your luck too far in planning the mañana baby. There's no magic cut-off point to circumvent trouble. Just remember there is a simple equation between aging and pregnancy. The longer you wait, the more difficult it is to become pregnant, and the greater the possibility of complications.

Fortunately many career women can become pregnant and have normal babies in their 30s. But obstetrics is based on batting averages, and older women, like aging baseball players, are more likely to strike out.

Drugs in Pregnancy

The French believed that no foreign army would ever penetrate the Maginot Line. But this myth was shattered by the sudden invasion of the German army in World War II. Doctors also clung to a myth for years; they believed the human fetus was protected from a foreign environment by the placental barrier. This fallacy was destroyed by the thalidomide disaster in the 1960s. The drug penetrated the placental sac and caused havoc in the normal developmental growth of the fetus. Now there's concern that too much coffee, too much alcohol, and excessive use of painkillers, tranquilizers, and antibiotics may also violate the natural protective covering of the baby.

Teratogenicity is the scientific term for the capacity of a drug to induce congenital abnormalities. But researchers now believe that some drugs may also cause functional behavioral problems later in life, and that pregnant women must realize that virtually all drugs cross the placental barrier to some degree.

Women should think seriously about the use of drugs long before they become pregnant. Major teratogenic effects start during the early weeks of pregnancy, perhaps even before some women suspect a pregnancy. Some delay the medical confirmation of pregnancy for weeks. In the meantime they continue to consume dangerous chemicals and carry on other bad habits.

Is coffee consumption a questionable habit during pregnancy? Doctors remain cautious about implicating this common beverage. But caffeine is under suspicion. In 1977, Dr. B.J. Van den Berg reported low birth weights in babies born to mothers who drank more than seven cups of coffee a day. Another researcher, P.S. Weatherbee, found that 15 of 16 women who consumed eight cups a day suffered more miscarriages and stillbirths. They also reported a similar risk in the wives of men who drank large daily quantities of caffeine.

Depending on the method of brewing coffee, as much as 300 mg of caffeine are consumed in one cup of coffee. Currently there is no convincing evidence that caffeine is teratogenic in humans. But prudence dictates that women who are either pregnant or contemplating pregnancy should use caffeine sparingly.

They should also think twice before drinking too many martinis. We know that the fetal alcoholic syndrome occurs in the offspring of chronic alcoholic women. These babies are born with small heads, facial abnormalities, mental retardation, and other growth deformities. Now researchers are sounding a new warning. They claim that doctors were too preoccupied with alcoholism in the past. It's their contention that alcohol, even in smaller amounts, can also cause behavioral teratogenesis, an abnormal change in the learning process and intelligence.

No one knows if there is a safe level of alcohol consumption during pregnancy. Evidence suggests that pregnant women who consume three or more alcoholic drinks a day are placing a baby at risk. This seems a reasonable conclusion. After all, it's been proven that just one ounce of vodka is sufficient to decrease fetal breathing.

Suppose a fetus could be granted one wish. It would request a non-smoking mother. Women who smoke are less likely to breastfeed a baby. Others may not have a child to nurse. Stillbirth deaths of smoking mothers are often coded as "death due to unknown cause," but there's good reason to suspect that these babies may have died of asphyxiation. Babies need a steady supply of oxygen, just like the rest of us. But carbon monoxide in smoke causes a significant reduction in the oxygen-carrying capacity of the blood. Studies show that smoking also causes "smoker's placenta." The afterbirth becomes larger in an attempt to pick up more oxygen from the mother, but this adaptation also makes the placenta thinner and more likely to separate prematurely from the uterine wall.

Nicotine also crosses the placental barrier with ease, triggering an increase in the baby's heart rate, an escalation of blood pressure and changes in the baby's muscular and nervous tissue. No woman should smoke during pregnancy.

The magic word during pregnancy should be "avoidance." One report reveals that 65 percent of pregnant women take painkillers at some time during pregnancy. But few pains of pregnancy justify the use of a mild painkiller. Tranquilizers and antibiotics are also widely consumed during pregnancy, but there is little knowledge of the possible teratogenic effects of these drugs.

The Bible gave sound advice to pregnant women 2,000 years ago. Judges 13:7 says, "Behold thou shalt conceive, and bear a son; and now drink no wine nor strong drink, neither eat any unclean thing." Will women ever learn to follow that sage advice?

What About Home Birth?

How do you answer the question of home birth? It's one I face every now and then in my office, often posed by well-meaning mothers. I've listened to all the heated rhetoric from both sides of the issue. I've read all the reports. I know what I'd like to say to young couples who ask for advice. But how to get the message across about this new trend without sounding dogmatic and hidebound? I've finally reached the conclusion that a film crew is the only way to provide couples with a convincing argument.

No wonder couples are confused. One noted professor has commented that home births are as safe as or safer than hospital deliveries. Another prominent authority says all evidence is strongly against home birthing. So who do you believe?

Home births have always been associated with the United Kingdom and Scandinavian countries. Nearly half the births in England used to take place in the home. Now it's under 2 percent and is rarely seen in Sweden.

Is this progress? The home enthusiasts say no. They contend that hospitals offer a cold, dehumanizing environment, that a warm home atmosphere aids labor, that women have the right to choose the location of childbirth, that home births bind families together, and that doctors should get in step with this modern trend.

But most doctors maintain it's madness to return to the old way. A former president of the American College of Obstetricians put it bluntly: "Should we stand idly by while American women rediscover risks forgotten by their grandmothers?" Some doctors have simply refused to attend a home delivery, and licensing bodies in some parts of the country have forbidden them to do so.

The debate on how women should deliver a baby can reach ludicrous proportions. For instance, one of London, England's, major hospitals recently put a ban on natural childbirth. The reason? One woman in labor demanded that she be allowed to remain on all fours instead of on her back. The midwife refused to assist until the patient assumed a more traditional position.

The subject of childbirth seems to be vulnerable to all kinds of theories today. I have great empathy for women in throes of labor. Does it really matter if a woman in labor wants to remain on all fours? Or even hang from a chandelier if this position eases her discomfort and helps the progress of delivery?

A film crew could settle this argument. A picture is still worth a thousand words. Couples could see what doctors face—not one single birth experience, but a whole range of them. It would be an eye-opener for those who maintain adamantly, never having seen one, that childbirth is a normal physiological process.

A film might first capture the beauty and serenity of a home birth, the joy of baby's first cry, the look of happiness on the faces of parents. All this without the clutter of fetal monitors and other threatening medical equipment that accompany hospital births.

But there might be a few unexpected surprises for the uninitiated. Doctors often look like they've been covering the Beirut war after an especially bloody delivery. Or like drowned rats when the fetal sac bursts unexpectedly. That warm and cosy bedroom at home may look like a disaster area on occasion.

Home birth advocates would also see the other, more frightening side of the picture. A young mother who hemorrhages suddenly when the placenta or afterbirth refuses to separate from the uterine wall. Now the normal calm is shattered when the participants realize there is no blood available to combat the shock. Lighting is poor and proper instruments absent. As is the anesthetist who must put the patient to sleep quickly so the placenta can be removed or a severe laceration repaired. Like flying, obstetrics, too, has its moments of sheer terror.

A film would reveal other occasional catastrophies: The look of apprehension on the doctor's face when he finds the umbilical cord caught in the vagina, cutting off the baby's oxygen supply; the dawning of the knowledge that the baby may die before a caesarean section can be performed. Time is never on the patient's side when complications strike. Nor is it possible to screen all patients from all potential hazards.

Dr. Sean McDonald of Prince Edward Island agrees. He says, "There's no comparison. I know what I prefer, and when you have done both, the only place is the hospital. You only have to look at tombstones in the graveyard to see how many babies died during childbirth in the past."

Diana, Princess of Wales, recently sought the safety of a London hospital rather than the comfort of a medical suite at Buckingham Palace. Possibly she's a student of history, and knows the old saying, "Those who do not remember history are destined to relive it."

11

Gynecology

Why Douche?

It's small wonder that women are confused about the safety of the birth control pill, or question whether estrogen causes cancer, or if too many hysterectomies are being done, when doctors can't agree about the simple douche. Some insist that it's a potentially hazardous procedure. Others are equally convinced that routine douching is of great benefit. Who is right and what should women do?

Differences of opinion are always refreshing. One astute businessman put it bluntly, "If I have two men on my board who think alike, one is unnecessary." It's a sound point if you're wheeling and dealing in the business world, or trying to find a cure for cancer.

But surely doctors should be able to agree on the simple matter of douching. It should take 10 seconds to give it a nod of approval or throw it out. Either way would at least put an end to the confusion of the female consumer.

Why are patients so surprised when I suggest it's desirable to douche? Some have been told by other doctors that douching washes away normal bacteria in the vagina. Others have heard that it causes infection. And often I hear them say, "Isn't it better to let nature look after it?"

Does this theory hold water? I can see how Leonardo da Vinci or Galen hundreds of years ago might have questioned its use. But today, when doctors are transplanting hearts and kidneys, this is medieval thinking. I wonder, for instance, whether these doctors ever brush their teeth? Wouldn't that also wash away normal bacteria? I think most of us would agree that nature does an inadequate job of dental hygiene.

Some of my colleagues have said to me, "You don't advise an enema every few days, so why subject the vagina to this routine?" They're quite serious when they propose this analogy. But is it reasonable to compare the rectum to the vagina? I don't think so.

Women should remember that although gynecology concerns only a small part of the anatomy, that part produces many of their problems. On an average afternoon most gynecologists offices are full of women, a good many of whom are suffering from common pelvic problems. Discharge and infection have always been at the top of the list.

It's easy to see why this is the case. Childbirth often leaves the cervical opening into the uterus torn and inflamed. Intercourse also results in some common vaginal infections. Other troubles can be picked up in a contaminated swimming pool or an unsanitary bathtub. Sooner or later most women contact vaginal infection or complain of an irritating discharge of one sort or another.

I frequently see women who have suffered from annoying discharge for years. They've been to several doctors and tried a variety of pills and creams without help. Some have a problem that requires additional treatment. Others simply have a large amount of normal discharge. No one has ever suggested douching, which promptly cures many of these patients.

I believe that douching is just another way of improving personal hygiene. I admit that douching with a teaspoonful of white vinegar added to a quart of lukewarm water won't solve all vaginal troubles, but it could ease the workload of doctors by preventing some common and bothersome problems.

An increasing number of physicians are advising patients to douche. But doctors face one persistent complaint when recommending this method of feminine hygiene., Douching has always been messy and inconvenient. I think that's why so many women reject it.

American women have a better deal than Canadian women. Several years ago in the book, *On Being A Woman*, I mentioned a new, revolutionary douche kit. It's called Portabiday and, like any new idea, it's amazing no one thought of it sooner. It consists of a long plastic handle with a sponge at one end which is dipped into cleansing solution prior to insertion. It's compact, easy to store, and handy to pack for a holiday.

The Portabiday is the most convenient method to date for good personal female hygiene. Regrettably, most Canadian women have never heard of this kit because of inadequate promotion. At the moment Portabiday is available only in the U.S.

Pap Smears—How Often? How Effective?

Should women always agree with the medical experts, the ones who say it's a waste of time and money to have an annual Pap smear if you are in the low-risk category for cancer of the cervix? Or is this a trade-off between dollars and lives?

In 1976 the Walton Committee and the American Cancer Society advised women that yearly Pap smears were not required under certain conditions. A woman with two consecutive normal smears after 18 years of age needs a Pap smear only every three years until age 35. After 35, if the smears remain normal, then screening once every five years was adequate until age 60. The Pap smear could then be discontinued if there had been normal smears up to that time. Annual smears were recommended only for women in the high-risk group.

I've never agreed with this advice. For one thing, I have a high index of suspicion about tests of any kind. Like the CAT scanner and ultrasound, the Pap smear is not infallible.

Pap smears may fail to pick up malignant cells for several reasons. The doctor may have placed too much vaginal discharge on the glass slide, obscuring abnormal cells. The technician who examines the slide may be suffering from a severe migraine headache. Or the discharge simply didn't contain any of the malignant cells. Human error, whether in a jet plane or the reading of a Pap smear, has the potential of coming into play. But should this happen during testing one year, the chances are extremely small it would occur again the next year.

Also, during my lifetime I've seen too many cervical cancers that should never have happened. Women who had normal smears for many years became careless. A few years later a smear shows a malignancy that should have been diagnosed much earlier.

Dr. Diane Crocker, Professor of Pathology at the University of Tennessee, shares this view. And she recently presented some shocking findings to the American Society of Clinical Pathologists. Dr. Crocker reported on 430 cases of cervical cancer. Of these cases 150 women had normal Pap smears one to five years before the diagnosis of invasive cancer. The average interval between the normal smear and the discovery of cervical malignancy was 2.6 years.

Another disturbing fact emerged. Cervical cancer, we've always been told, occurs more often in women of low socio-economic status, where there is early sexual activity and poor hygiene, and in those who have had several pregnancies. But Dr. Crocker's research revealed that advanced cancer of the cervix was seen even among women who were not considered to be in the high-risk group. These women had developed cervical cancer in three years or less after normal smears had been reported.

She also had a special warning for women in other countries. For instance, in Canada, where the screening rate had decreased, the mortality from cervical cancer has increased 25 percent over a 10-year period. And in England and Wales, where the same relaxed approach prevails, deaths from this malignancy have doubled.

Here's my advice: Remember that this type of cancer could be wiped out if all women had an annual Pap smear. Moreover, don't stop this precautionary test once you reach 60 years of age. One third of Dr. Crocker's cases with prior normal smears developed cervical cancer at or after the age of 60. In another study done at St. Vincent's Hospital in Worcester, Massachusetts, an 82-year-old woman developed cancer of the cervix which spread to other organs; her Pap smear had been normal three years earlier.

Dr. Crocker charges that there's been "a trade-off of dollars for lives" in the recommendations of the Walton Committee and the American Cancer Society. Regardless of whether her critical verdict is right or wrong, it will result in the premature and unnecessary deaths of some women. Make certain you are not one of them.

How serious is it when a Pap smear is reported as abnormal? Today this test has become an integral part of the annual gynecological examination. For the majority of women the result reassures them that cancer isn't present. But for others its result causes alarm, sometimes needlessly. So patients should know a little about this test and what it is looking for.

The rationale for the Pap smear is quite simple. Cells from the cervix (the opening into the uterus) are constantly discarded into the vagina. They're easily seen when vaginal discharge is studied under the microscope. If cancer of the cervix is present, malignant cells are also present in the vaginal discharge.

Women who are told the Pap smear is abnormal usually react in the same way as those who discover a breast lump. They immediately conclude a malignancy is present and disaster has struck. But this is rarely the case if a Pap smear has been taken every year.

Cancer, like most things, isn't white one day and black the next. Cars don't suddenly collapse on the highway, but fall apart bit by bit. Nor does hair suddenly turn grey. Body cells act the same way. It's impossible for them to be normal one day and cancerous the next. Instead they go through a definite series of changes on their way to malignancy.

The Pap smear is an extremely sensitive test which detects minor changes in the cervical cells. Not all abnormal changes are related to cancer. Vaginal infections, inflammation of the cervix, or a chronic lack of the female hormone, estrogen, can cause abnormalities in cells similar to changes seen in cells on their way to becoming cancer. Once the infection is cured or these other problems treated, the cells and the Pap smear return to normal.

But suppose the abnormal smear is not related to any of these problems? What is done depends on the classification of the smear. For example, the majority of patients will have mild cellular changes. These women are advised to have a repeat smear in a few months. Some minor changes in the cell structure will revert to normal without any treatment.

But smears showing moderate to severe changes cannot be ignored. The Pap smear informs doctors only that abnormal cells are being thrown off from the surface of the cervix. It provides no indication whether there are abnormal cells beneath the surface. Or from what part of the cervix the cells originate.

The mandatory next step is a colposcopic examination. The colposcope, like a microscope, magnifies the cervical area several times. Doctors can take biopsies of suspicious areas. These small bits of tissue are then analyzed by the pathologist. What follows depends on the severity of the change, the age of the patient, and whether future pregnancies are desired.

Patients with moderate or severe changes can often be cured by cryosurgery. This painless office procedure freezes the cervix and destroys abnormal cells. Healing takes about six weeks. Pap smears are then repeated in a few months to see if abnormal cells have been replaced by normal ones.

But doctors may also recommend conization when severe changes are present. During this hospital procedure, a cone-shaped piece of tissue is removed from around the entire cervical opening. It removes any further areas that might contain abnormal cells, as well as providing additional tissue for pathological examination to make doubly certain an early cancer isn't present. This approach conserves the uterus for future pregnancy, and even if a small surface malignancy is discovered, no further treatment may be needed.

Hysterectomy is advised under certain conditions. A surface malignancy may be present and some patients feel more comfortable having the whole uterus removed. Or occasionally the Pap smear will continue to show worrying changes after conization has been performed. Prevention is still better than cure. There is no point in passively watching cellular deterioration year after year until a cancer is full grown.

Cystitis: Why Some Women Shouldn't Take Baths

Maurice Chevalier often said, "Vive la différence!" when referring to the female sex. I'd heartily agree that a woman's body has some endearing features, but the Great Creator made at least one slip in designing the female anatomy. He or She gave it a very short urethra, the tube that carries urine from the bladder to the outside, making the bladder easily accessible to infection from a variety of causes.

"Honeymoon cystitis" is often a bride's first encounter with cystitis. Frequent intercourse at this time subjects the bladder to more than the usual trauma. And the bladder is just like any other part of the body. Overactivity may cause tennis elbow, sacroiliac pain, and cystitis.

But the urethral opening endures more than sexual trauma. It's located at an extremely vulnerable and busy location. Since it's situated at the top of the vagina, infections from this area and the rectum can easily spread to it.

Childbirth may also cause bladder misery. The stretching of the vagina during childbirth frequently results in the bladder's falling down. A bladder that has dropped doesn't empty completely, and the remaining urine acts much like water in a stagnant pool. It is more easily infected.

Less frequently the bladder is affected from another direction; there may be an obstruction blocking the normal outflow of urine from the kidney, which triggers infection. Or a kidney stone may precipitate the trouble. But whatever the reason, an infected kidney pouring bacteria into the bladder must be treated before recurrent cystitis can be cured.

Usually people who rush to the bathroom simply have a full bladder. Those with cystitis also complain of burning on urination and a dull, dragging pain in the low abdomen. If the bladder is badly inflamed, the urine will be bloody, and often the desire to urinate produces little urine.

How doctors treat cystitis depends on whether it's a first or a recurrent attack. Initially culture and sensitivity studies are done on the urine. Since many different bacteria cause cystitis, it's important to determine which type is present. The laboratory can also find out which antibiotic is best suited to combat the infection. Lucky patients may never have a second attack after a single course of antibiotics.

Patients with recurrent attacks must have kidney x-rays and a cystoscopic examination to explore the inside of the bladder. Sometimes an operation is needed to remove an obstruction or a kidney stone or repair a fallen bladder.

What other means will prevent recurrent cystitis? I don't have 10,000 cases to prove this point, but I've been impressed with one clinical fact over the years. It's that women with this problem often take baths rather than showers.

Ring-around-the-collar may be a problem for some males, but that ring-around-the-bathtub is a more devastating one for women. I've never heard of a research study that analyzed the bacterial content of bath water. But I'd bet it would incriminate dirty water as one cause of recurrent cystitis. Women who have access to a shower should avoid the bathtub.

I'm impressed with another fact that's often overlooked in treating this disorder. Elderly women with cystitis have frequently taken every available antibiotic. They've received repeated x-rays and cystoscopic examinations. But no one has either done a pelvic examination or been impressed by an inflamed, dry, aging vagina that's crying out for estrogen.

Cystitis and senile vaginitis coexist for one good reason. The lining of the lower part of the urinary system is the same as the vaginal lining. So giving estrogen to restore the vaginal lining to its normal thickness also has a beneficial effect on the urinary tract.

Here are some other preventive measures: Urination following intercourse helps to remove bacteria that may have been thrust into the urethra. Moderation in the frequency of intercourse and the use of alcohol will also decrease the chance of an attack. And although not all physicians agree, I believe regular douching is desirable.

Should Women Hold a Purse in Their Teeth?

How do women maneuver over a public toilet? Like other males, I've often wondered what a candid camera would record. This week my curiosity ended. A woman reader from Portland, Oregon, presented me with a fascinating scenario. The picture she describes of women in this predicament is comical, but it also demands male sympathy and poses some interesting medical problems.

The topic arose over a bridge table. One of the reader's friends had remarked that the only sex education she received from her mother was, "Don't ever sit on the toilet in a public washroom." Everyone laughed and admitted they'd been told the same thing. The suspicion created in the child had lingered, and they all still obeyed their mothers' advice.

The letter asked, "There are millions of women out there balancing on high heels, pantyhose straining at their knees, purses clutched tightly in their teeth while hovering over the toilet bowl. We'd love to know if it's all necessary?"

Should women improve their balancing act? If they sit and relax, are they going to leave with venereal disease? Or at least some annoying infection? And what exactly is it that lurks threateningly on the edge of that toilet seat?

It all reminded me of a professor in medical school. I was accompanying him on hospital rounds one day and came upon a patient he was treating for repeated bouts of gonorrheal infection. Although obviously a lady of questionable reputation, she complained that she must have picked up the disease on a toilet seat.

The professor was a quick-witted fellow. He had also become bored with this story. He speedily replied, "That is a rather strange place to have intercourse." He explained that there was a million-to-one chance of contacting VD on a toilet seat. These germs are quickly destroyed on contact with the air.

But before you drop your purse and relax, there are other facts to consider. Doctors are often criticized for being able to transplant hearts and still be unable to cure the common cold. It is equally amazing that we know so little about common vaginal infections.

For instance, tens of thousands of women suffer from trichomonas. This microscopic, protozoan organism produces annoying discharge and irritation. We know it can be transmitted by sexual intercourse, and I suspect it can also be caught from swimming pools and infected bathtubs. It, too, is killed quickly by contact with air. But toilet seats are often wet and may harbor the culprit. I'd still chew on my purse.

It's a rare day when I don't see a patient with fungus infection. Most of these patients are circumspect about hygiene. Some haven't been within a mile of the neighborhood swimming pool, nor have they been in someone else's bathtub. So how did they pick it up? I don't know. And I haven't seen any research papers that can answer that question. Until I see evidence of a specific breeding ground, I'd keep improving my balancing act.

While hovering over the toilet seat, I'd keep in mind other infections. There are several bacterial infections that cause bothersome vaginal discharge and itching. Doctors are also seeing more women with herpes of the vulva. This is a tough diagnosis to accept, because there's no known cure.

There's another reason to brush up your hovering technique. Doctors see more women today with warty growths on both the outside and inside of the vagina. This disease is caused by a virus, and repeated treatments or hospitalization are needed to cure it. I've never sneaked into women's washrooms to culture the toilet seat. But I'd bet the virus is there. And who knows whether the last patron had a draining boil on her posterior?

I hesitate to mention the next point. The last thing I want to do is create a nation of toilet seat hypochrondriacs. But there's a proven fact to consider. One enterprising researcher did invade the men's room. He discovered that when males urinate, the spray can be detected three feet away. Now I know how high the spray rises over Niagara Falls. But who knows about a woman's toilet bowl? Perhaps more than just the seat is the problem. We may have to redesign the mechanism.

My knowledge of women's washrooms is limited. But over the years I've cast a jaundiced eye at the state of men's washrooms. Some look like they haven't been cleaned since the War of 1812. And it never fails to amaze me how often people fail to flush the toilet.

I wish it was possible to end the contortions and anxieties of women hovering precariously over toilet seats. But if I were a woman I'd prepare for the public washroom with care and precision. I'd hope the Almighty had endowed me with strong teeth and good coordination. I'd hate to drop my bag on most washroom floors. I'd do some exercises to improve my balancing act, possibly read a book about Houdini to learn how to maneuver in tight compartments. And learn how to squat comfortably three feet above the toilet bowl.

And if I lost my balance? I'd rush home, take a hot shower, boil the pantyhose, and keep on practicing my balancing act. Good luck.

Time for a Change in Underwear

A reader recently complained to me, "It's impossible to buy a pair of undies that doesn't fit like a second skin. The same goes for girdles. A gartered girdle for women who wear stockings is now almost unobtainable." She made a strong plea for manufacturers to give back our old, loose underdrawers.

Second-skin pantyhose may make you look like a ballerina, but nature never intended the female anatomy to be hermetically sealed. The body was designed to breath. Today's pantyhose and panty girdles confine and suffocate the pelvis. This in turn leads to a variety of female problems.

During the warm months of summer, I always see a rash of skin problems. Obese women are particularly prone to a disease called intertrigo, which occurs wherever skin surfaces rub together. Perspiration is retained due to inadequate circulation of air. Gradually debris collects in deep creases, and the skin becomes soft and macerated. Women can be chronically plagued by this condition. They often make repeated visits to a doctor, complaining of itching and irritation. For good reason. Intertrigo can spread to the inner thighs and lower abdomen. The entire vaginal area may become a fiery beefy-red.

Some women have to endure more than pantyhose intertrigo. For instance, the chronic deterioration of skin decreases its resistance to infection. It becomes an ideal breeding ground for bacteria. An intense increase in itching may also be due to fungus infection.

Women frequently confide how difficult it is to tolerate the itching. After all, it's not an area one can scratch in public. But scratching in private often causes skin abrasions and a secondary infection. Occasionally hair follicles on the vaginal lips develop a pustular eruption, or painful boils appear. And if the patient has diabetes, these problems are intensified.

There are several dos and don'ts if you suffer from pantyhose intertrigo. First of all don't treat yourself. Or listen to the next-door neighbor's latest remedy. Patients frequently arrive on the doctor's doorstep after over-treatment with a variety of chemicals and ointments. Some in desperation have used Lanacaine ointment. This is like putting a blanket over a roaring fire. Moreover, some women become sensitive to Lanacaine.

Simple measures are usually the best therapy. It's vitally important to clear up vaginal infections first. You're fighting a losing battle if discharge continues to bathe an already inflamed skin. And once infection is eradicated, regular douches will help to keep the vagina healthy.

Pantyhose intertrigo will usually respond to simple hygiene, calamine lotion, and drying powders. But don't use powder while the skin is still wet. This causes caking and further itching.

The cure for some cases can turn into a physician's nightmare. Some women will momentarily be relieved by antibiotic ointments. Others will be helped by a combination cortisone-antibiotic cream. Still others in the menopausal years require an estrogen cream to alleviate the symptoms. Yet some patients return to the doctor several times a year with recurrent pantyhose problems. Or wander from doctor to doctor seeking relief from this trouble. There is only one solution for these women. Obese patients must lose weight, and all women need a new improved style of pantyhose.

Endometriosis: Stringing Males Up by the Thumbs Might Prove a Point

What a pity women can't string their husbands up by the thumbs, then when they complain, tell them the pain is simply psychological. It would be just retaliation for husbands who accuse wives of feigning painful intercourse. Often, in fact, they've been suffering for years from severe endometriosis. Internal bleeding is a common finding during pelvic examination. But it's occasionally undetected by doctors, and then chauvinistic husbands compound a missed diagnosis.

During normal menstrual periods, the endometrial lining inside the uterus bleeds. Endometriosis occurs when some of this lining escapes outside the uterus. Pieces of it become attached to the ovaries and other pelvic structures, looking much like a surgical transplant.

How this happens is debatable. Some gynecologists believe it's due to retrograde bleeding through the fallopian tubes. For instance, if a hysterectomy is performed during a menstrual period, it's occasionally possible to see blood coming out of the tubal ends. Others think the endometrium is transported by either small lymphatic channels or blood vessels.

Career women who postpone pregnancy are more prone to develop abnormally displaced endometrium. It also bleeds during a period. But the blood is trapped within the pelvic cavity and triggers menstrual peritonitis. This inflammatory reaction causes scarring of the female organs, bowel, and other structures. In some cases blood-filled cysts develop that can reach the size of a grapefruit or larger.

Women with endometriosis complain of increased menstrual pain and heavier bleeding, and may have trouble getting pregnant due to scarring and adhesions of the fallopian tubes. And since the most common site of endometriosis is at the end of the vagina, painful intercourse is common. In fact, sexual relations can be almost unbearable.

Minimal endometriosis is an elusive diagnosis. In some instances it's necessary to insert an optical instrument, the laparoscope, into the abdomen to detect the problem. But doctors can usually feel the tender endometriotic lumps at the end of the vagina.

Husbands should realize that endometriosis is an unpredictable disease. Like a forest fire, it sometimes burns out without need for treatment. The menopause also automatically cures endometriosis. Lesions melt away when there's less female hormone to stimulate abnormally displaced endometrium.

What is advised depends on the patient's age, the severity of the symptoms, the extent of the disease, and the prospect of further pregnancies. For women desiring a pregnancy the hormone progesterone is given in increasing doses for several months. This stops the periods, with the result that lesions often simmer down. Other drugs, such as danazol, are helpful in select cases. Sometimes pregnancy occurs following this therapy.

Surgery is reserved for women with severe symptoms and extensive disease. On occasion endometriosis has totally destroyed the female organs. Then the surgeon has no choice but total hysterectomy. For women desirous of more children, a more conservative operation is done. Gynecologists perform what's called a presacral and uterosacral neurectomy. In this case the surgeon cuts these two nerves which transmit painful sensations to the brain. This relieves pain but has no effect on sexual sensation or orgasm. If a pregnancy follows, there may be no pain in the first stage of labor.

During an operation to conserve the female organs, the surgeon also cauterizes areas of endometriosis that are scattered throughout the pelvic region. If endometriosis involves the ovary, part of the ovary is removed. The uterus is suspended in its normal position if adhesions have pulled it backward to the spine. This type of surgery relieves symptoms in about 70 percent of cases.

Complete hysterectomy, with removal of tubes and ovaries, is chosen for extensive disease and when the patient has completed her family. There is no point in this case in performing an operation with "maybe" results.

But don't fall into this trap if you've completed your family: Never assume that total hysterectomy is planned. Remember that some surgeons are compelled to preserve the uterus at any cost. The surgeon may change his mind at the time of surgery and leave the uterus in place. This could leave you with a "maybe" result, opening the door to hysterectomy in a few years. In the interim chauvinistic males will still believe the pain is in your head.

Vaginitis: What Treatment?

I'll be bold enough to suggest an eleventh commandment for doctors. It reads, "Thou shalt always examine the patient and never use shotgun therapy when treating vaginitis in women." This commandment, seemingly logical enough, would prevent months or years of needless suffering for both the patient and her husband.

Vaginitis, a common malady, is an inflammation of the vaginal wall. And it sometimes takes the cunning of Sherlock Holmes to detect the cause. For instance, one patient, a 19-year-old girl, was unable to walk because of extreme swelling of the vaginal area. But laboratory studies revealed no reason for her disability. Later she admitted trying to bleach her pubic hair with ammonia.

On occasion a desperate call to Inspector Clouseau seems the only recourse. In one case of vaginitis I tried every cure on a recurrent fungus infection, but to no avail. Finally as a last-ditch effort, I asked the patient, "Do you have animals in the house?" That's when I discovered that she had a female dog, and the plot began to unfold. This well-dressed immaculate woman had trained her dog to urinate in the bathtub when she was away for the day. A veterinarian confirmed that the dog had vaginal fungus infection.

Scotland Yard isn't needed to diagnose most cases of vaginitis. Yet often these infections go undiagnosed and cause persistent trouble. Some women suffer so much inflammation that intercourse becomes impossible. These are not life-threatening problems, but they can take much of the joy out of life.

Trichomonas infection causes the most vaginitis. This unicellular organism is about the size of four white cells. It is extremely fragile and dies within a few seconds when exposed to a dry surface. But inside the vagina trichomonas has the resistance of a lion. Some women with this infection are totally unaware of its presence. But the majority of patients complain of a profuse, irritating, malodorous discharge.

Vaginitis is also caused by fungus infection. It, too, produces discharge, but in contrast to trichomonas the irritation is usually intense. Often the lips of the vagina swell as well.

Bacterial infection attacks the vagina as it does other parts of the body, but there is a vital difference here. A quick look at a sore throat tells the doctor something is wrong. But bacterial infections of the vagina do not cause an acute reaction. They can be present for years without detection. Or if detected, they can be misdiagnosed and patients receive a variety of medications with no effect.

But why the need for another commandment? The reason is that I hear so often the same story from patients. They've been troubled by discharge for years and received a variety of medications from the family physician. But he's neglected to do a pelvic examination, or hasn't taken vaginal smears during the office visit. This makes as much sense as the mechanic who fails to open the hood of a car when something's wrong with the motor.

There's another reason for a commandment. Some physicians use shotgun therapy. Vaginal creams containing a mixture of drugs are available that attack several types of infection. So doctors tend to prescribe this combined package rather than do a pelvic examination. This shortcut works occasionally, but shotguns won't stop charging elephants. And this method is less likely to cure recurrent vaginitis. There's no substitute for making a specific diagnosis by vaginal smear, then using the appropriate drug.

Vaginitis has strong social overtones. A woman may be fearful of mentioning the annoyance to her husband, thinking he may be suspicious of her activities. Others worry that the husband has been with another partner. And repeatedly women complain, "I always take such good care of myself. Why do I have this trouble?"

For the young generation there is a simple reply. Today's freewheeling sexual mores have triggered a huge increase in vaginitis. The birth control pill may have liberated women from the fear of unwanted pregnancy, but some pay a price for this freedom.

Couples must not make the error, however, of blaming each other. Vaginitis has been known to result from a dirty bathtub, a whirlpool bath, a swimming pool, an unclean toilet seat, the use of antibiotics, or the presence of diabetes. And as long ago as 1966 the American Medical Association bluntly stated, "Oral contraceptives are now known to enhance vaginal fungus growth." Tight-fitting pantyhose or jeans may also be responsible. But in many cases the specific cause is still a wild guess.

My advice to women with this problem is simple. Don't accept a shortcut for recurring vaginal infection. Never accept a prescription without an internal examination. And cast a wary eye at the doctor's examining room that has no microscope for vaginal smears. After all, the doctor would react the same way if a mechanic didn't open the hood of his car.

Premenstrual Syndrome and the Plea of Insanity

"Members of the jury, have you reached a verdict?" the judge asks.

"We have, your Honor. We find the defendant not guilty of committing murder, possessing a dangerous weapon, setting fire to the house, abusing her children and assaulting three policewomen. We agree with the precedent set by Smith and Adams that the defendant is suffering from the premenstrual syndrome and therefore not responsible for her actions."

This may be a slight exaggeration of what may soon become a familiar verdict in North America. If I were the Godfather, I'd watch this development with great interest.

The premenstrual syndrome (PMS) affects a large proportion of the female population. The usual symptoms are swollen, tender breasts, fatigue, headache, skin eruptions, crying spells, depression, and cravings for sweet and salty foods. But can it trigger aberrant behavior and criminal acts?

Dr. Katharina Dalton thinks so. She's associated with the Premenstrual Syndrome Clinic at the University of London, England. Her report on three convicted women, which recently appeared in the British journal, *The Lancet*, has far-reaching ramifications for Canadians and Americans.

One 28-year-old woman had been convicted 26 times for theft, writing threatening letters, and finally a fatal stabbing. During her prison term she slashed her wrists, broke windows, and attempted to drown herself.

Another 18-year-old girl shaved her head and eyebrows, ate weedkiller, set fire to the house, and tried to strangle herself. Still another threatened to kill her grandmother, escaped from a hostel, and threw a knife at a man.

These women pleaded diminished responsibility for the crimes. All received lighter sentences from the judge. One charge was reduced from murder to manslaughter. The judge accepted the explanation that the accused were suffering from premenstrual tension when the crimes were committed.

PMS is now accepted as justification for crimes committed in the United Kingdom. In France it is used by lawyers as grounds for a plea of temporary insanity. And there may soon be a test case in Michigan. Imagine the field day attorneys will have using this alibi for clients. It boggles the mind.

Can PMS be held totally responsible for such criminal acts? And, if so, can it be prevented? Dr. Dalton believes these women suffer from a deficiency of the female hormone, progesterone. She states that regular injections of this hormone will stop aberrant behavior.

Doctors on this side of the Atlantic have varied reactions to this use of progesterone. Louis Keith, Professor of Obstetrics and Gynecology at Northwestern School of Medicine, says the treatment is unorthodox, but may prove to be reasonable.

Cynthia Cooke, Assistant Clinical Professor at the University of Pennsylvania School of Medicine, is more positive. She accused U.S. male doctors of xenophobia and sexism when they condemned Dr. Dalton's research. North American gynecologists, she insists, place too much emphasis on surgery to solve female problems. Too many women wander from doctor to doctor seeking relief from PMS. And most often they get either a pat on the head or a tranquilizer.

Other gynecologists are less enthusiastic about progesterone. Georgeanna Seegar Jones, at the Eastern Virginia Medical School, hasn't found the hormone effective. In fact, she believes it aggravated the symptoms of some patients. Her theory is that PMS is due to an overly active nervous system. The best treatment? Learn to live with your nervous system.

Most women don't require medication for PMS. Some need diuretics to rid the system of excess fluid. Other patients obtain relief from aspirins, birth control pills, and relaxation exercises. But results are hard to evaluate, as some women are helped simply by placebos or sugar pills.

What's my advice to judges? I think the courts should cast a skeptical eye at this excuse. I'd agree it's safer to tease a lion than some women with severe PMS. But the act of stabbing a victim is criminal behavior, not PMS. I fear Dr. Dalton's theory is a dangerous one, and lawyers will seize it as a defence for violent anti-social behavior.

What an opportunity this would create for the Mafia! They could hand out all illegal assignments to their wives. It wouldn't matter if they were charged with arson, murder, or liquidating a dozen policemen. The wives could plead PMS and that they forgot to take their progesterone.

Painful, Lumpy Breasts Can Be Cured

How would males react if their testicles became lumpy and painful several days every month? Or were tender to touch day after day? Would they be satisfied when a female doctor reassured them the pain was not due to cancer? I doubt it. Male chauvinists would more likely scream to high heaven and demand more research to rid them of this misery. Yet male physicians forget the golden rule when treating women with painful breasts.

Dr. Earl Peacock, Jr., wrote, in the journal *The American Surgeon*, "Reassurance that it is not cancer will allay all fears and the pain becomes bearable." Tens of thousands of North American women with fibrocystic disease of the breast might wish him painful testicles and the same advice.

Fibrocystic disease of the breast affects one out of every six women between the ages of 35 and 50. The extent of this problem varies from patient to patient. Some breasts have hard areas of thickening with small BB shot masses scattered throughout them. Other patients have very discrete cysts, like marbles, that are easily felt.

Painful breasts are common prior to the onset of the menstrual period. Fibrocystic disease accentuates this normal tendency. But as the disease progresses, discomfort often becomes a daily affair. Even the slight pressure of clothing or bedding triggers pain.

This problem was first described by Sir Ashley Cooper in England 100 years ago, but he had no idea what caused the trouble. It wasn't until 1970 that Dr. Bernard Eskin of the Medical College of Pennsylvania in Philadelphia threw some light on this disease.

His work revealed that patients with underactive thyroid glands had an increased incidence of breast cancer. Later another study in Japan also confirmed this association. Eskin carried his research a step further. The thyroid gland requires iodine to function properly, so Eskin placed rats on an iodine-free diet. This produced precancerous changes in their breasts. He then discovered that if he also gave these rats estrogen, this caused greater cyst formation in the breasts. When iodine was later restored to their diet, breast architecture returned to normal.

Does the same thing happen in women? Russian scientists reported several years ago that potassium iodine produced favorable results in 78 percent of patients with cystic breasts.

But the strongest evidence that iodine is beneficial originates at Queen's University in Kingston, Ontario. Dr. William R. Ghent, a professor of surgery at the university, has given iodine treatment to over 1,000 women with fibro-cystic disease of the breast. He reported to the Cancer Society meeting in Toronto in 1983 that 88 percent of his patients had been cured by this technique. He is hopeful that it won't be too long before nearly 100 percent of women with fibrocystic disease of the breasts can be helped.

It's been my contention for years that women have received shabby treatment from some male surgeons in the management of fibrocystic disease and cancer. In the past some women with breast malignancy have been subjected to a radical operation when a lesser procedure would have produced the same results.

I've seen other female patients who have multiple, needless scars on their breasts from the repeated removal of small lumps. These incisions could have been prevented if the doctor had thought of the needle instead of the scalpel. We know that 85 percent of all breast lumps are benign, and many of these are cystic. It's a simple procedure to insert a small needle into the lump to determine if it is a solid mass or a cyst. In the event the mass is cystic, the fluid can be removed, the cyst collapses, and the patient gets a good night's sleep knowing that it's unlikely that cancer is present. I've been aspirating cysts for years and have no reason to regret it.

Currently I'm following Dr. Ghent's procedure to ease the pain and tenderness of fibrocystic disease. Fortunately there are few side effects to iodine, and results to date are very rewarding.

12

Estrogen

"Would you prescribe estrogen for your mother?" a reader from Kamloops, B.C., recently asked me. It's a good question. We all have a healthy respect for our mothers. No doctor would advise her to take aspirin, estrogen, or any other drug if it were dangerous. But he also wouldn't withhold medicine if it would prevent some problem. Is there a sensible way to take estrogen? And what advice would I give my mother?

Estrogen had a disastrous year in 1976. A Boston study linked the hormone to cancer. The report became an instant headline around the world. The obvious question entered my mind: Should I tell my mother to throw away the estrogen?

But many of the facts didn't add up. Women were suffering from cancer of the uterus and breast long before researchers discovered estrogen. I have visited many areas of the world where doctors rarely prescribe this hormone. But women in these countries were still dying from these diseases.

There was another reason why I didn't place a quick call to her home. The Boston findings were based on figures, not on test-tube research. And it's been proven repeatedly that there are three kinds of lies: Lies, damned lies, and statistics.

Now a recent report in the prestigious *New England Journal of Medicine* confirms my fears about statistics. The authors say that women on estrogen have 20 chances in 1,000 of contracting uterine cancer. Since tens of millions of women in North America have taken estrogen for decades, we should have a raging epidemic of this disease. But where is it? Cancer of the uterus remains a relatively rare problem. Only 60 in 100,000 women develop this trouble.

How should women handle the estrogen question? First of all, don't become a victim of the estrogen backlash. Remember that scare headlines never tell the whole story. What happens is that patients who need this hormone fail to receive it.

Estrogen has many useful purposes. For example, it may be needed to increase the thickness of the vaginal lining before a hysterectomy or vaginal surgery. Some patients may require it to relieve troublesome hot flushes or intense irritation at the vaginal entrance. Painful intercourse may also continue unless estrogen cream is applied to a thin, ulcerated vaginal lining.

So don't quickly raise an eyebrow if the doctor suggests estrogen. There's a chance you'll leave the office without this hormone. Why? Because he may be having a particularly tough day with no time for a detailed discussion about the merits of estrogen. Then there's another human factor that comes into play. Doctors are tiring of fighting alarming headlines. If you frown too much, he may take the path of least resistance and agree with you.

I think there's a simple message for doctors and their patients. You have to use common sense when taking estrogen, just as you do when swallowing aspirin, antibiotics, or other drugs.

Luckily one-sided headlines have some advantage. They help to restore good sense and bring people back to basic principles. For example, there's no point in taking more estrogen than you need. The dosage must be tailored to each patient.

Doctors also advise taking estrogen three weeks on and one week off. They believe it reduces the risk of abnormal bleeding and cancer. Possibly they're right. But if troublesome symptoms occur on the week off tell your doctor. After all, ovaries normally produce estrogen every day. So I've always questioned the wisdom of this estrogen holiday following the menopause.

What should post-menopausal women do when bleeding occurs while they are taking estrogen? There are several important don'ts to remember. Don't assume it's normal and due to the change of life. Don't wait to see if it will happen again. Don't quickly conclude it's due to either cancer or the estrogen. Rather, make a speedy appointment to see the doctor. He'll arrange to have a D and C (scraping of the uterus) done.

Let's suppose he doesn't suggest it, that he agrees that the bleeding is due to your age or estrogen. Don't ever accept this wait-and-see attitude. The bleeding could be due to a malignancy. Putting off a D and C could be a fatal move. Be sure to get another opinion.

What about my mother? She's a speedy 89 and still going strong. I told her to take estrogen over 25 years ago, and that's still my advice. Maybe estrogen prevented her from getting osteoporosis, a thinning of the bones, possibly saving her from a few broken bones and other problems. I'll let my readers know if I ever tell her to throw away the estrogen.

Aside to Internists

Some medical specialists cause needless sexual problems. They don't expect Englebert Humperdinck to sing with a sore throat, yet they expect women to enjoy sexual intercourse with an inflamed vagina. These doctors would scream like hell if I took their heart patients off digitalis. Yet they're continually taking my patients off estrogen. It's time they bought a speculum and gave females and their husband a break.

Several times a year I fume at internists. They would be the first to fire the garage mechanic who didn't bother to look under the hood of their ailing automobile. But they believe their training permits them to ignore this fundamental approach in the treatment of female problems. And they give advice without doing an internal examination.

Here's an example of what happens to some women. I've prescribed the female hormone estrogen to relieve menopausal hot flushes or to treat annoying vaginal discharge or to relieve severe pain during sexual contact. The reason for avoiding sex is obvious on examination. The inflamed vaginal walls look as if they've been scraped with sandpaper. Within a week estrogen cream relieves such symptoms.

Later, I see these patients again and the condition has recurred. Some women stop taking estrogen after reading a sensational article linking the hormone to cancer. Others take the advice of poorly informed friends, or fail to renew the prescription. Still others are bluntly told by an internist to discontinue the medication. And 99 percent of the time, the doctor hasn't bothered to do a pelvic examination.

When I encounter this situation, one thought enters my mind. How many other women in Canada are caught in this same trap? There must be thousands.

Why would a specialist in internal medicine advise against estrogen without first inspecting the vagina? There are several reasons. First of all, internists are human like everyone else. In recent years controversy has whirled around this hormone. Some physicians, like patients, develop a psychological bias against any form of estrogen treatment.

Specialists in internal medicine spend their days studying electrocardiograms, treating failing hearts, diseased kidneys, and migraine headaches. The female organs are as far removed from their field of vision as the oil fields of Saudi Arabia. If the thought ever crossed their minds to perform a pelvic exam, they'd have to borrow a vaginal speculum.

Doctors who routinely do pelvic examinations are keenly aware of the fact that ovaries age like other organs. Menopausal ovaries produce smaller amounts of estrogen, resulting in the thinning and ulceration of the vaginal lining. Doctors refer to this condition as senile vaginitis. But it also occurs in young women who have had a hysterectomy with removal of both ovaries. Today the aging vagina is the most overlooked gynecological problem in North America.

What should you do when a second specialist tells you to stop taking estrogen but doesn't do a pelvic examination? Patients are naturally reluctant to question professional expertise, and many have also had doubts about hormones. Most women don't have to be told twice to throw the pills down the drain.

But don't fall prey to this bias. The doctor has already shown that his expertise is a trifle frayed at the edges by omitting the vaginal examination. He wouldn't treat Humperdinck's sore throat without looking at it. The same horse sense applies to vaginal ailments.

A female physician would have good advice for you. She'd know these symptoms might be the result of a lack of estrogen. They could also be triggered by bacterial, fungus, or trichomonas infections. She'd seek the advice of a colleague who didn't use a crystal ball for diagnosis.

My advice for internists? Remember that the aging vagina requires estrogen to prevent and cure painful intercourse. That the hormone has proven it retards thinning of bones once the menopause begins. That there is evidence it offers protection against heart attacks and strokes. That it can be a useful adjunct in treating chronic urinary infections and the dry eye syndrome. That there have been millions of women on estrogen for over 30 years. Surely there would have been a raging epidemic of malignancy if this hormone caused cancer.

Can we make a deal? I won't interpret electrocardiograms if you won't take my patients off estrogen. This compromise could save women and their husbands considerable trouble. But if you don't agree, please at least buy a vaginal speculum.

Will Lack Of Estrogen Make You Rob the Local Bank?

Gifford-Jones has often been roasted, lampooned, and rapped on the knuckles by courtroom lawyers. But last year I finally had a chance to tackle these brilliant attorneys on my own battleground. A Canadian judge had publicly become an instant expert on the menopause. A 48-year-old woman complained in his courtroom that a man had stood across the street, exposed himself, and urinated in front of her. But she lost the case because the judge ruled that the menopause made her evidence unreliable.

That's when I had my day in court. I wrote a column giving the legal profession a short course on the menopause. I hoped that Canada wouldn't be the first country to draft a "menopausal clause" into the statutes. That would be a tough job even for lawyers.

What would be the magic age when unreliability begins? Some women start the menopause at 35, others at 55. Then how would you handle a 30-year-old woman who has had a hysterectomy? If the surgeon left in one ovary, would she be only half reliable? And how would attorneys treat a 45-year-old woman who was taking the birth control pill? Would the estrogen in the pill make her a *bona fide* witness? Equally important, should a 60-year-old judge take a shot of the male hormone testosterone before he reached a verdict? What's sauce for the goose is sauce for the gander.

The directors of the Criminal Lawyers Association said they were going to study the verdict of the menopausal woman versus the man who exposed himself. The Attorney General also planned to do some research work on the matter. But it seems they still haven't completed their homework.

Now a defence lawyer has blamed shoplifting on the menopause. He contended that his client was unable to fully appreciate what she was doing due to menopausal depression. To add insult to injury, a psychiatrist got up from his couch, testified as an expert witness, and agreed with this hypothesis. The woman was found guilty, but the judge granted her an absolute discharge. It would have made some famous professors of gynecology roll over in their graves.

Perhaps the time has come to appoint a government inquiry to separate menopausal fact from fancy. At least we need a short primer on the menopause for psychiatrists. If we don't do something, the legal fraternity and many others will be left with the wrong information on this common problem.

Gynecologists would agree that some uptightness may accompany the hot and cold spells of the mid-life change. But in 20 years of clinical practice I've never seen it cause sufficient agitation to start a woman on a robbing expedition. Or to hijack a plane, or be unable to determine whether or not a man was exposing himself in public.

The legal profession has done its best to complicate its own field so none of us know what's going on. There's no need for them to do the same thing with medicine. Unlike their writs, the menopause is a simple problem. The ovaries age, like every part of the body, and eventually they are unable to produce sufficient quantities of estrogen. It's the lack of this female hormone, estrogen, that causes the bothersome hot and cold spells.

Menopausal women who bypass estrogen are more likely to get frayed nerves at this particular stage of life. But it's also easy to overplay the role of estrogen in relieving uptightness. In most instances the tension is due to marital problems, teenage children, and empty nest syndrome, and the fact that life is passing by. Men have also been known to suffer similar symptoms at this point for the same reasons. Why blame the menopause for a variety of troubles that are unrelated to it?

It is ludicrous for judges, attorneys, and psychiatrists to associate the menopause with criminal activities. Normal women don't rob stores, nor do they suddenly lose their eyesight or their sense of propriety about men displaying their wares in public.

Failure to carry this message to the law courts will result in an odd brand of justice. If you take estrogen the judge might believe your story. But if you plan on robbing the neighborhood bank, stay away from the hormone. It's a great alibi to explain that you didn't really know what you were doing.

How Estrogen Can Ruin a Vacation

How many women this year will have their vacations spoiled or cut short because they developed chills and hot flushes even before packing their bags. Their doctors prescribed estrogen, which quickly stopped bothersome symptoms. Yet in the rush of his office, he forgot to warn the patient how estrogen can ruin a holiday.

Women who journey south are particularly vulnerable to this trouble. The majority are either at or past the menopause. They need estrogen, but receive it at the wrong time. Estrogen, like a new pair of shoes, is best tried while you're at home.

Why do women start estrogen just prior to a trip south? Psychologically, people like to see the doctor before leaving on a holiday. Sometimes it may spot a problem. A 65-year-old woman will be found to suffer from senile vaginitis and require estrogen to restore the vaginal lining to normal thickness. Others will have menopausal symptoms that necessitate this hormone. Still others are simply at the age when some doctors believe it's a sound idea to start estrogen replacement therapy (ERT). Most women are grateful for the treatment. Yet after their arrival in Florida, a few will develop post-menopausal bleeding. A good many will worry about the possibility of cancer. And the fun is suddenly gone.

What has happened to cause the bleeding? Estrogen has numerous effects on the body. One purpose is to stimulate the inside endometrial lining of the uterus during the reproductive years. At this time the endometrium is highly responsive to estrogen, and it becomes thicker in preparation for a possible pregnancy.

Later on in life the withered endometrium does not react as much to estrogen. Yet on occasion it still has enough get up and go left in it to produce spotting or outright bleeding.

What should you do if this happens in Florida? It basically depends on the timing. If it occurs a couple of weeks before you return home, you may as well wait to see your own doctor. But send him a letter explaining what has happened. This should ensure a prompt appointment on your arrival back home.

But if the bleeding occurs several weeks before a scheduled return, there are two choices. You should fly north immediately or see a Florida gynecologist. It may result in a wasted trip home. Most likely a D and C will reveal a benign polyp or fibroid or merely prove that the bleeding was due to estrogen stimulation of the endometrium.

Yet much better to cut a vacation short than delay for months, only to discover that a cancer has been present. Never, never procrastinate by waiting to see if the bleeding will occur again. It's an approach that could cost you your life. And if your own doctor or the one in Florida tells you the trouble is due to estrogen, without an examination or a D and C, get another opinion.

Is there any way to prevent ruining a Florida vacation? There's no 100 percent method, but you can trim the chance by following a few simple rules.

Remember never to pack new shoes or new drugs in your suitcase. If you're having menopausal symptoms or just want a checkup, see the doctor long before you head south. In the event you require estrogen, there's ample time to adjust the dosage to your own needs. Taking the lowest possible dose will decrease the risk of abnormal bleeding.

It's also wise not to push the doctor towards estrogen if you've suddenly read an article stressing the benefits of ERT. If you haven't needed estrogen for the last 10 years, you can do without it at least until after your return from Florida.

Women with senile vaginitis who need treatment can temporarily sidetrack the oral estrogen tablets or the intra-muscular injections by using local estrogen cream. Since only a small amount is absorbed by the body, post-menopausal bleeding is rarely encountered. Then they can start oral estrogen on returning home.

13

Female Surgery

What Every Woman Should Know About Hysterectomy

Should you or should you not have a hysterectomy? Every year this burning question enters the minds of 800,000 North American women. For some the operation will be a life-saving procedure; for others, it will merely end a chronic annoyance. Yet about 300,000 women will help the surgeon pay the office rent, purchase a new Cadillac, or finance a Caribbean vacation. Hysterectomy is now big business, which nets doctors over half a billion dollars a year. With so much money involved it's important that patients ensure the surgeon is thinking about their health, rather than his bank account.

How can such a staggering number of women go astray when the consumer has become more and more skeptical of surgery? There's no doubt that the red light does flash on in many women's minds when the doctor suggests this operation. But even if it goes on with the intensity of a neon sign in downtown Las Vegas, about one woman in three gets trapped into having a questionable hysterectomy.

One reason is that it's difficult to beat people at their own game. The plumber and TV repairman often give the doctor a thumping. Nearly everyone strikes out with the lawyers, and not many get the jump on bankers. Having the alarm buzzer go off is one thing, but it's another matter to prove the doctor right or wrong. Today too many women give the surgeon the benefit of the doubt.

There are several pitfalls. Hysterectomy has a notorious track record for presenting women with conflicting opinions. A trusted friend says she has never felt better since the operation. Yet another one vehemently condemns the surgery because it has failed to relieve her complaints. The uninformed patient wonders who she should believe, and it becomes a no-win situation.

The operation itself conjures up many unanswered questions. Some women have the wrong impression of what a "total hysterectomy" signifies, and are sometimes surprised and annoyed when they find out. Others wonder whether or not the ovaries should be removed and whether the menopause starts after the surgery. Still others are confused about the need for estrogen, particularly since recent reports have associated this hormone with cancer.

Hysterectomy has become so much a part of the North American scene that it often appears to be the "in thing" for some women. They seem to believe that sooner or later they'll require the surgery, so why put it off?

There's also more to the problem than the needless hysterectomy. Some women get a double whammy. They undergo a "Knick-Nack-Ectomy," in which the surgeon removes part of an ovary, a tube, suspends the uterus, or cuts the nerves that go to this organ. It's a desirable approach in some circumstances; however, it's also possible to end up with two needless operations rather than one. Other patients who have a hysterectomy done may have an ovary left in when it makes no sense to do so.

The "hysterectomy backlash" is another hidden pitfall, and it can cost some women their lives. Patients with a curable precancerous lesion sometimes sidetrack the surgery because they have read a melodramatic magazine article censuring the operation. Remember that each year 500,000 of these procedures are done for *bona fide* reasons.

To try to alleviate the confusion, I've written a book called *What Every Woman Should Know About Hysterectomy*. I hope that it gives the consumer an updated, both-sides-of-the-coin appraisal of this common operation and also provides insight into areas that are neglected in discussion of this topic. For instance, some women who enter the hospital for this procedure return home without having it performed. They had prepared themselves psychologically for the surgery and had never dreamed that something else would be done. A knowledgeable patient can circumvent this problem.

This consumer approach to hysterectomy will be criticized by some physicians. They will say that a little knowledge is a dangerous thing and that women cannot understand these complex matters. That's nonsense. Most problems in gynecology are straightforward ones and all you need is common sense to make the right move. For example, it takes little mental acuity to conclude that the new trend towards hysterectomy sterilization is fraught with needless dangers. Or that some bleeding problems are best handled with patience, hormones, or a D and C rather than quickly jumping towards a hysterectomy.

There are also sensible guidelines that help to determine which women have an increased chance of developing emotional troubles following the surgery.

Some critics of this book will say that most surgeons do good work and that hospitals have controls that spot knife-happy doctors. That's only partly true. Otherwise there wouldn't be 300,000 needless hysterectomies every year. A thinking, informed patient is still the prime protection against questionable surgery. Moreover, in evaluating surgeons, remember what Pubilius Syrus said in 50 B.C. "He hurts the good who spares the bad."

Should Ovaries Be Removed During Hysterectomy?

Most women never ask the surgeon what he plans to do with the ovaries at the time of hysterectomy. In some cases the question is of little importance.

Women over 50 will most probably have them removed. Patients in their early 30s will leave the operating room with the ovaries intact unless they are diseased. But there are situations where what is done with the ovaries can be of vital importance. Leaving the decision entirely to the surgeon can backfire on the patient later on in life.

Women in their late 30s and early 40s are in an "ovarian no-man's land." Some gynecologists will invariably remove both ovaries even if they appear normal, which results in an instant menopause. Other gynecologists routinely leave them in if they appear to be normal. It's reasonable for patients to wonder why doctors vary so much in their approach.

One day I was operating with a distinguished gynecological surgeon. He was in a rather philosophical mood and pondering this question. He admitted that often what he did with the ovaries depended on his recent experiences with patients. If he had just watched a woman die from ovarian cancer, he removed them. If he hadn't seen this tragedy for some time, he was more inclined to leave them in.

This is an honest appraisal of what may be in the back of the surgeon's mind. It's not a very scientific approach. But since that time nothing has happened to make it an easier, more cut-and-dried decision.

Why do some surgeons bend over backwards to save the ovaries? They see no reason to remove ovaries that may continue to produce adequate amounts of female hormones for many years. Why produce an artificial menopause that will require the taking of estrogen pills or injections long before they would normally be needed? Retaining ovaries is more convenient and less expensive.

If you ask about the possibility of ovarian cancer developing, they have a standard reply. They say if you're worried about this possibility, why not also amputate breasts for the same reason. Ovarian cancer is not a common malignancy compared to breast cancer.

How do other gynecologists defend their liberal removal of ovaries? They think that comparing the ovaries to breasts makes little sense. You can't replace breasts with anything else. Conversely, ovarian hormones are readily available and relatively cheap.

They agree that most women who have ovaries left in do not develop cancer. But why take that chance when it's easy to swallow a hormone pill every day? Moreover it's impossible to do a hysterectomy without some interference of ovarian blood supply. Some remaining ovaries therefore develop pain or become cystic. Why take the chance of needing another operation later on?

There is no guarantee that the ovaries of a 38-year-old woman will continue to function for another 10 years following a hysterectomy. Hot flushes may start within a year or two. Estrogen will be required, and useless ovaries have been left in place.

At other times retained ovaries may adhere to the end of the vagina, causing pain during intercourse. If the discomfort is severe, an operation may be required to remove the ovaries. I've also known patients who have undergone hysterectomy and assumed the ovaries had been removed. Later when a cancerous ovary developed it was a double blow when they thought this could never happen.

Don't ever assume that the ovaries will be removed if the surgeon says he intends to do a total hysterectomy. He may mean total removal of the uterus and conserving ovaries.

Some women have strong psychological feelings about being more of a woman if the ovaries are left in place. If that's the case, let your doctor know how you feel before the operation. Other women are happier if they are told the best ovary will be left in. The main thing is not to wake up to surprises. You can only prevent this by a frank, open discussion with the surgeon prior to the operation.

Whether or not to remove the ovaries will continue to be a contentious issue for many years. But one thing is not debatable. Regardless of what has taken place pre-operatively, the findings at surgery take precedence over everything else. The surgeon may have the best intentions of preserving ovaries, but following the incision find this would not be in the best interests of the patient. A good surgeon would never allow his hands to be tied so that he could not have the final decision.

Should Women Have the Right to a Hysterectomy of Convenience?

Do women have as much right to a hysterectomy as to a teeth-straightening procedure. A U.S. doctor reporting in the *American Journal of Obstetrics and Gynecology* thinks so. His study shows that 78 percent of patients felt better following hysterectomy, 70 percent had less inconvenience, 54 percent had more energy, and 38 percent a better sex life. So does hysterectomy on demand make sense? Or is it sheer surgical madness? How can the consumer sift the assets and liabilities of this surgical technique?

How do women talk themselves into this operation? There's no doubt that the monthly period is a nuisance, particularly for the increasing number of women entering the business world. And it's easy for male surgeons who make the final decision to "pooh pooh" an inconvenience they've never experienced.

Consider the case of a 25-year-old career woman who is irrevocably dedicated to a childless life. Of the next 20 years, 5 of them will be spent in menstruation. Since most women flow heavily the first day of a period, she will frequently have anxious moments before an important meeting or speech. Traveling becomes more difficult for her. Male doctors would listen to these problems with more sympathy if they were born with a uterus.

No doubt a "demand" hysterectomy would save some lives. After all, you can't die from cancer of the uterus if that organ has been removed. A shrewd businesswoman might even use her calculator to demonstrate some facts. About 100 out of every 100,000 hysterectomies end in a fatality. But more than 100 of this same number will develop a uterine malignancy.

The operation would also remove fear of unwanted pregnancy. There would be no need for messy contraceptive creams. Or worry about complication from an intra-uterine device. Or the potential hazards of the birth control pill. One cannot completely discount the radical views of this American doctor.

But how do you talk yourself out of this surgery? A good starting point would be to question women who have had a hysterectomy of convenience. One in 10 say they are unhappy with the results, and one in six would not recommend it to friends. It appears that such surgery does not solve all female problems.

I'm sure that some patients find that hysterectomy also has some inconveniences. Some suffer from severe abdominal distension and vomiting after the operation. It's no fun to have a stomach tube draining a paralyzed bowel for several days.

Others get more than they bargained for when the incision becomes infected. In some instances this merely prolongs the hospital stay. But in others the infected wound leaves a hernia which requires a second operation to be repaired.

There can be other unpleasant surprises. A few patients may be rushed back to surgery to control post-operative bleeding. The occasional woman develops phlebitis. A very rare one either dies or comes close to it from an unexpected clot in the lungs. And some patients are left with a chronic annoyance. Vaginal hysterectomies, in particular, may shorten and scar the end of the vagina, resulting in years of painful intercourse.

What is my advice about hysterectomy of convenience? Never forget the procedure is a major operation and that sometimes minor surgeons are performing it. This is true in this country where large numbers are done by self-trained family doctors.

In general it's wise not to seek out potential trouble. Never amputate the arm if cutting off the finger will accomplish the same end. Or jump onto the operating table if there's no immediate need for it.

I agree that the female consumer has rights, possibly even the right to a hysterectomy if she's willing to accept one risk over another. Maybe that decision will save her life from cancer. But rights also entail responsibilities. Irresponsible hysterectomies may make some women wish they had spent the time on a Caribbean vacation.

What would I advise a female member of my own family? I'd have grave reservations about hysterectomy of convenience. How could I ever forget my advice if a major complication resulted? I'd always remember that inconvenience never killed anyone.

The Lumpy Breast

Most women don't understand the breast. To many the discovery of a lump automatically means that a cancer is present. Others believe that it's mandatory to remove every breast lump by surgery. Still others fail to realize that the normal breast undergoes considerable change during the monthly cycle. These misconceptions cause many sleepless nights. They also set the stage for questionable operations as apprehensive patients push surgeons to remove one lump after another.

Finding a lump is not always the prelude to major surgery and the loss of a breast. Sixty-five to 80 percent of these lumps are benign. Some are hard, fibrous growths. Others are single cysts. But most lumpy breasts are due to a condition called fibrocystic disease (FCD). It affects about one in every six women between the ages of 35 and 50. That's why it's important to know the facts about this common problem.

Why do cysts develop in the breast? Doctors are not sure, but they have some hunches. For instance, cystic disease occurs during a woman's reproductive life when there is an abundance of the female hormone estrogen. Then when the menopause begins and estrogen production decreases, the cysts tend to disappear. It's for this reason that doctors believe estrogen plays some role in this disorder.

FCD varies from patient to patient. Some breasts have areas of thickening with small hard BB shot masses scattered throughout them. Other women have more discrete cysts, like marbles, that are easily felt.

Painful breasts are common prior to the onset of the period. The presence of FCD accentuates this normal tendency. Some women find it terribly annoying and require diuretic pills to remove this excessive fluid that helps to cause the discomfort.

How do surgeons separate these benign lumps from the cancers? Some physicians believe that all lumps should be removed. They argue that it's impossible to differentiate the good from the bad unless they're examined under the microscope. Since no surgeon wants to miss diagnosing a malignancy, this approach has considerable merit.

But cutting out every lump that forms also has its problems. Some breasts are loaded with them. It would necessitate excising the entire breast to examine every lump. The doctor therefore has to use his clinical experience in deciding which, if any, of the lumps should be removed. In addition new techniques such as mammography can help him to pinpoint suspicious lesions.

Some doctors, therefore take a more selective approach to breast lesions. They believe that some women who have multiple scars on their breasts could have been handled in a less traumatic way by aspirating these cysts. It's a simple and painless procedure. The skin over the lump is frozen with a local anesthetic and a small needle is inserted into the mass. If this test shows that the lump is solid, you must change the ground rules and remove it. But if the mass collapses as the fluid is withdrawn, it's a good sign that the lump is benign. It's like handing the patient a million dollars when she can no longer feel the worrisome mass.

One third of the surgical professors who were polled believed this was a good way to treat some lumps. The others were concerned that a small cancer in the wall of the cyst could be missed by the aspiration technique.

No one would deny that a doctor can miss a malignancy by relying on this method for some lumps. Yet doctors have reported a large series of cases where it has been used without regret. For example, one study revealed that of 2,000 aspirations only one malignancy was discovered from examination of the fluid. No cancers subsequently appeared. And one patient had 78 cysts treated over a six-year period.

S me doctors will remove the first cyst to prove it's not a cancer and to relieve the patient's fears. But if other cysts form, they'll resort to the aspiration technique. This can save multiple breast scars, needless hospital admissions, and the risk of a general anesthetic.

Physicians may differ on how they handle some breast lumps, yet they all agree on one point. Never be your own doctor in treating this problem. Rather, make a prompt appointment for an expert opinion.

Radical Mastectomy or Lumpectomy?

Women face two psychological traumas when told breast cancer is present. First, they are all struck by the fear of the disease. The ultimate loss of a breast is the second terror. But is radical removal of the breast really necessary? Do the results justify this mutilation? Does a simple lumpectomy offer the same chance of cure? How do women separate fact from fiction when confronted with this problem?

I've recently discussed this dilemma with a variety of eminent doctors. One point stands out. Most women are not aware of the basic facts when they submit to a radical mastectomy. If given complete information, many patients would opt for a lesser operation.

How do radical surgeons defend this drastic procedure? They claim that the breast, the underlying muscles, and the lymph nodes in the armpit must all be removed. Why? Because cancer cells may have already spread to these areas. If they're left intact the patient will die.

Some surgeons are quite vehement in justifying this approach. One says, "If you fail to do it, you're playing Russian roulette with a patient's life."

These doctors condemn the lumpectomy advocates as "faddists." They stress that, to date, experience with lesser operations is too limited to draw any sound conclusions. They also remind us that 6 out of 10 cancers already exist in other sites of the breast. Perform a lumpectomy and these cancer cells are missed.

Conservative surgeons, on the other hand, say that mutilation and psychological stress are all in vain. Look at mortality figures for the last 50 years. In spite of radical surgery the cure rate for breast cancer has not improved. They say the reason is staring us in the face. If malignancy has already metastasized to the armpit, it's also spread to more distant parts of the body.

Their advice to radical surgeons is to stop kidding themselves. How can the scalpel excise malignant cells in the armpit which can only be seen by the microscope? In essence they accuse them of trying to close the barn door after the horse has escaped.

It's true, they say, that breast cancers often occur in several places in the breast. But this also happens in the other breast. If radical surgeons were consistent in their thinking why wouldn't they remove both breasts?

The conservative surgeons bring up another interesting point. It's known that 30 percent of men over 50 and 50 percent of those over 60 also have microscopic evidence of cancer in the prostate gland. But few of these men die from prostatic cancer. Possibly these other cancer cells in the prostate and breast are not true malignancies. Conservative thinking demands that surgeons confine their efforts to removing the main cancerous growth and using other means to destroy the distant metastases.

Who do you believe when faced with this decision? There is no easy answer to the question. But when there is such profound disagreement among surgeons, women should at least have some say in what operation is done.

Don't forget that the cure rate appears to be about the same with all types of surgical treatment. This is because both sides cure the malignancy confined to the breast. Once the cancer has spread, survival rates drop for all surgeons.

More and more studies indicate that it usually makes little sense to submit to radical surgery and its complications. Many patients are left with a deep psychological disfigurement. Moreover, there is often painful swelling and scarring that may limit the future use of the arm.

There seems to be a new theme in the air—that surgeons should upgrade their thinking and confine their efforts to removal of the obvious growth. Then a decision can be made as to whether or not radiation should be given. Since an increasing number of small cancers are being diagnosed early by mammography, this theme seems to make sense.

But is lumpectomy swinging too far in the other direction? Some surgeons who shy away from the radical removal of breast, muscle tissue, and lymph glands still believe the whole breast should be excised. Yet other prominent surgeons say that a lumpectomy is sufficient for about 50 percent of all breast cancers.

In reaching a decision, it's often a wise idea to take a look at other countries. For example, in England, Scandinavia, and France the radical mastectomy operation is rarely done, and their results are equal to those in the U.S.

Hopefully the days of radical breast surgery are on the way out. This in itself may have another indirect benefit. Women may seek medical attention earlier when they realize breasts can be saved.

Should the Breast Be Rebuilt After Cancer Surgery?

Some women who undergo breast removal for cancer are given the choice of an artificial implant. But a very high percentage never receive such an option. Why is this the case when loss of a breast triggers so much sexual, psychological, and marital tension?

General surgeons are, in most cases, reluctant to advise such a possibility. A heated debate of this issue is currently running between general and plastic surgeons. Women should be aware of both sides of the argument.

General surgeons frequently contend that silicone implantation makes it difficult to detect recurrence of cancer. Others fear that a second operation to insert the device may reactivate dormant malignant cells.

Some surgeons reveal a cloak of male chauvinism. They insist on telling post-operative patients they should be grateful to be alive and well. Or that the surgeon who is concerned about restoration of the breast may skimp on the initial operation in order to leave some form. And that, for the sake of appearance, some patients die needlessly.

But in recent years there's been a trend to more limited surgery of the breast. Radical removal of the entire structure has not improved the survival rate. Simple removal or lumpectomy in selective cases is performed more frequently today. This means that more women may now be good candidates for reconstructive surgery.

Plastic surgeons suggest that women should be given a choice before the breast is removed. This offers an additional benefit. Increased opportunity for a reconstructed breast may decrease the delay in seeking help. Many women procrastinate too long about seeing a doctor when a lump is found in the breast.

Does an artificial or rebuilt breast affect the patient's chance of survival? Dr. Jerome Urban of Memorial Hospital in New York recently replied to this question, "I do not believe there is any reason to expect that reconstruction with a silicone prosthesis would have any effect on increasing recurrent disease." Other surgeons agree that it is a very remote theoretical possibility.

What should women do who face the worry, anger, and psychological trauma of losing a breast? Remember that a sense of timing is vital in many things in life. It's also important for women contemplating reconstruction of the breast. "Do not do today what you can sensibly put off until tomorrow" is a wise approach to this type of cosmetic surgery. For instance, 85 to 98 percent of local recurrences of breast tumor occur within two years. Delaying the implantation of a silicone device until this period is over seems a reasonable move.

Delay is helpful in another area. It gives women the chance to think it over.

Some patients lose their zeal for the operation in time. The final realities of the situation may not be as severe as initial expectations. And they become accustomed to wearing an external prosthesis.

Women should be cautious on another point. Don't be tricked by current journalism on the subject. The suggestion that a new breast is available to all and the solution to all problems is irresponsible and misleading. Keep foremost in your mind that the breast can never be restored to normal. Plastic surgeons can create a breast, but it is always a synthetic one, and not necessarily a perfect match.

Women contemplating this surgery should do more than merely discuss the procedure with a plastic surgeon. They should also look at before-and-after pictures, or talk with a patient who has had the operation. This could determine the choice quickly. And it can also be of great help to the surgeon.

Some people mistakenly believe that plastic surgeons wield a magic scalpel. They want artistic perfection and are annoyed when the result fails to measure up to expectations. It's impossible for surgeons to live up to the standards set by some patients.

Yet, for other women, the chance to have a synthetic breast helps remove part of the fear of this surgery. For these, the breast remains a badge of femininity.

Some surgeons have suggested that we live in a breast-oriented society, that being able to wear a bikini is often more important than survival. But the breast's sexual significance is not a twentieth-century concept. Fascination with the female breast dates back to Biblical times. Jacques Thibault in 1893 summed up the feelings of many when he wrote, "A woman without breasts is like a bed without pillows."

The 100,000 North American women who face cancer surgery of the breast this year should be aware of their options. For some an artificial breast may be better than none at all. Others may decline a purely cosmetic second operation.

Patients Should Tell Some Surgeons How to Operate

Should patients ever advise surgeons how to operate? After all, it would be madness for passengers to tell a pilot how to land a jumbo jet, or instruct a plumber in the repair of a leaking pipe. It's much safer to mind your own business. But every year some women have two operations when only one is required. It happens because surgeons occasionally mix morality with medical judgment.

Here's a typical example of what can happen when a patient leaves all the decisions to the doctor. A 35-year-old woman came to my office accompanied by her 40-year-old husband. They couldn't believe a diagnosis they'd received in another city and wanted a second opinion.

Two months earlier, Mrs. X had been referred to a gynecologist for sterilization. He advised that the procedure shouldn't be done if there were any doubts about future childbearing. She was also warned that the operation could not guarantee 100 percent results.

This couple agreed to proceed under these conditions. They had four children and wanted protection against an unexpected pregnancy. They understood that such surgery cannot always produce perfect results. But they were stunned to learn that a pregnancy had occurred within a short time after the operation. Surely the doctor must be wrong, they insisted. And did I agree?

This couple were not in a betting mood. But if I'd been asked the same question in Las Vegas, I'd have been willing to give them an answer without benefit of an examination. I'd also be prepared to tell them something else they didn't suspect. And I'd bet ten-to-one odds I was right. I have no direct line to the Creator, and no special talents as a diagnostician. But I've learned something from seeing the same scenario played in my office time and time again.

I had little doubt that this patient was pregnant. She had not menstruated following surgery. She complained of morning nausea, breast tenderness, urinary frequency, and fatigue. Pelvic examination confirmed the diagnosis beyond doubt.

What had gone wrong? The patient concluded that the surgery was a success but the operation had been a failure. I knew better. My clue was the size of the uterus. Mrs. X had become pregnant a couple of weeks before the sterilization procedure was performed.

It's logical for women to ask how this could happen. How could a seasoned gynecologist miss the diagnosis? There's a simple reason, but you must be part physician, theologian, and philosopher to understand the answer.

It's both a lack of common sense and a carelessness prompted by fear that sets the stage for this complication. Some doctors have an unconscious dread of unintentionally interrupting a few-days-old pregnancy. They avoid this problem by neglecting to do a preliminary D and C (scraping of the uterus) before the sterilization. Doctors who fail to use this safeguard may eventually operate on a pregnant patient. There is no way to avoid this except by D and C. This is because pregnancy tests are unreliable in the early stage of pregnancy. Today's birth control methods are not 100 percent effective. And a woman who has not missed a period may still be pregnant.

It's a shattering experience when women come face to face with this useless result. They are usually well-motivated patients who approach parenthood responsibly. Many are looking forward to becoming grandmothers rather than mothers. Now they have to accept the trauma of another child or an abortion.

Can you avoid this pitfall? First, don't make the error of prematurely stopping contraception before sterilization. Women who are scheduled for this surgery often feel relieved psychologically. They see an end in sight to childbearing days and become careless about birth control.

There's only one sure way to circumvent this misfortune. Request the surgeon to do a D and C as part of the sterilization procedure. If he refuses, find another surgeon unless you live in a remote area where there's little or no choice.

There's another sound medical reason for doing a D and C at this time. Many patients who request a sterilization are in their 30s. This is a decade when the uterus is more prone to disease. A D and C may reveal an unexpected benign polyp, fibroid, or early malignancy.

Medicine and theology can be a spectacularly winning combination in times of stress. For the terminally ill patient theology offers more than chemotherapy and doctors combined. But if you're not careful, it can also lead to two operations rather than one.

"Zipper" Sterilization

An ingenious entrepreneur struck it rich when he invented the zipper. It's an effective, time-saving, and practical device for men's trousers and women's dresses. But some people are giving the zipper too much credit. They've come to believe that medical progress has created "zipper sterilization" for both sexes. Some patients will get their fingers burned on this philosophy. Why is this new microsurgery a potential hazard? And can Gifford-Jones's Law alert you to a new danger?

Vasectomy for men and tubal sterilization for women now rank third behind the pill and the IUD as contraceptive choices. This year about 160,000 Canadian women and 50,000 men will opt for these procedures. Unfortunately some of these people regret their decision.

Recently a new patient in my office was stunned and astonished. I'd just told her it was not a simple task to restore her fertility. The tubes had been severely damaged by laparoscopy cauterization, and I thought her chances of success were minimal following a complicated operation. I would not recommend it.

It's easy to see why many people believe we've entered the age of zipper sterilization. Too many articles have appeared in magazines and news items stating that new techniques can make sterilization a reversible procedure. A stitch here and a snip there sounds easy when you say it fast. But there's many a slip twixt the hand and the lip in this type of surgery.

Why? Because when plumbers join together two large drainpipes there's a chance of trouble. But fallopian tubes are about the size of a piece of spaghetti. The vas deferens is half that size. And the canal that runs through both is no larger than the eye of a needle. So miniature surgical plumbing of this kind is a tedious business, particularly when these structures have been damaged by sterilization.

Women face an additional hazard. Doctors in the past sterilized females through appendectomy-like incisions. The fallopian tubes were cut and tied, causing little damage to the remainder of the tube. Now increasing numbers of women are sterilized by laparoscopy. This optical instrument, similar to the periscope on a submarine, is inserted into the abdomen through a half-inch cut. The tubes are then cauterized, causing extensive injury to much of the tube. It's a major task trying to unzipper these tubes.

What about microsurgery? How has operating with a microscope changed the rules of the game? And why am I apprehensive about this new advance in surgical technique? If progress is good for General Electric, shouldn't it also be good for patients?

I'd answer with a big "yes" for some surgical operations. For instance, being able to look through the microscope during surgery has been a tremendous asset in repairing deaf ears. It's also a useful adjunct in eye operations, joining together small blood vessels, and in brain surgery.

So why do I answer with a resounding "no" when considering microsurgery to repair damaged fallopian tubes? I've stressed in previous columns a very basic point. It's that what is good for a doctor's family is also sound advice for other patients. And I would never advise a female member of my family to undergo a reversal operation.

Remember I said "female member." I wouldn't argue too strongly about a male member of the household. Does that imply I'm a male chauvinistic pig? It simply means that once again men get the better deal. Removing a blockage from the vas deferens just requires a small incision in the scrotum. If the operation fails, the loss is minimal. But to reconstruct the injured female tubes, a large incision is needed, involving greater danger and more pain. I don't believe the risk justifies the poor results.

You should also consider Gifford-Jones's Law before agreeing to microsurgery. This law states, "If surgeons have a spanking new instrument, they will always find patients on whom to use it." Surgeons who have spent time learning this technique won't want to keep the microscope in the closet.

What should female patients do who are considering a reversal operation? Don't forget that what seems sensible in headlines may appear less so from a hospital bed. It's possible an egg may never enter the tube at all. Or it may become stuck in an imperfect tube, causing ectopic pregnancy. You'll then face the additional trauma of an emergency operation to remove the pregnancy.

I'm not against sterilization. I believe men and women should have access to this procedure for a variety of reasons. But once the decision is made, I wouldn't look for the non-existent zipper. Good contraceptives are available today. Use them until you're 100 percent sure you want sterilization.

The Surgical File of Patient X

What would you do if the surgeon said, "I'd like to perform another operation on you. It isn't going to improve your health one iota. You may still have the same old symptoms. In fact the pain may get worse. It may mean more surgery in a few years time to cure you. But don't worry, it may also show us what's wrong." Faced with such frank remarks we'd all run for the hills and find another doctor. But patients do have such totally useless surgery. Here's why it often happens in Canada and the U.S., and how you can avoid this fruitless exercise.

One surgeon who performed such an operation is a Fellow of the Royal College of Surgeons. In addition he's a member of a prestigious Canadian clinic. It's proof that the right diploma doesn't necessarily mean common sense will be applied to surgical problems.

A 32-year-old woman had suffered for years from pelvic pain and abnormal bleeding. She had an operation to remove an ovarian cyst at age 20. It was followed by two caesarean sections. During the last caesarean she was sterilized. Later a fourth operation was done to excise part of an ovary. The patient's pain and bleeding problems continued to escalate after each operation. Finally in desperation she consulted a surgeon at one of this country's better known clinics.

A senior gynecologist decided to make a fifth incision. The operative note describes a gloomy picture. The pelvic organs were surrounded by adhesions. Loops of bowel and remaining ovarian tissue were rigidly adhered to the uterus. One ovary contained a large blood clot.

The surgeon decided to try the impossible to conserve the uterus. Bowel was dissected free from the uterus and adhesions were severed around the ovaries. The female organs were left intact. The result was predictable. The patient continued to have pelvic pain and bleeding. The surgeon remarked in a post-operative report. "This patient will probably end up with a hysterectomy in the future."

The patient was told a different story. She was advised it was wiser to preserve the uterus at her age and that the operation would ease her symptoms. He had added an interesting comment: Before a hysterectomy could be performed, her case would have to be presented to a committee.

Every year in North America thousands of questionable operations are done. Some are performed by family physicians without any formal training in surgery. Others, like this one, are undertaken by well-qualified surgeons.

But this case illustrates a special kind of needless surgery. For example, many people have unnecessary tonsillectomies, hemorrhoidectomies and gallbladder operations. Occasionally these procedures are followed by post-operative complications, but usually removal of the gallbladder or tonsils puts an end to surgery in that part of the anatomy.

Female pelvic procedures are too often repetitive. I see many patients who have had "Knick-Knack-Ectomies." One operation leads to another and still another. Eventually hysterectomy becomes the only way to relieve the patient's symptoms.

Granted, it's mandatory to conserve as much normal tissue as possible in young women or in those desiring additional children. But there are times when a surgeon should perform more definitive surgery. Women who are past the childbearing age are in this category. So are women who have endured several previous operations, and those who have completed their families or have been sterilized. To do anything short of a hysterectomy becomes a questionable approach.

Suppose this patient had been the surgeon's wife? Would he be annoyed at what was done? I think he'd be furious. He'd remind the surgeon that his wife had been sterilized. So why did he worry about doing a hysterectomy at age 32? She had endured four other operations; he should have suspected the large blood clot in the ovary was due to endometriosis, which would require a hysterectomy. His judgment was poor.

If you've suffered through several pelvic operations be careful about the next one. There's a good chance you need a hysterectomy rather than a Knick-Knack-Ectomy.

When to Get a Second Opinion

I recently startled a 40-year-old patient after an office examination. I said, "In your situation, you shouldn't believe me." The problem was that she didn't have any symptoms, but during examination I discovered a large fibroid tumor filling her pelvic cavity. It would eventually cause pain or heavy bleeding. I knew she needed a hysterectomy. But she would be convinced only after another opinion. When another consultant agreed with me, she would believe I wasn't a knife-happy surgeon, and she would then enter the operating room in a better psychological condition.

Every year thousands of people receive such an unexpected blow. For the first time in their lives they face major surgery. The physician's diagnosis may sound plausible. But they arrive home with lingering doubts. Should they get a second opinion? Would it save them from the scalpel? Or would it be merely a waste of time and money? There are some warning signals to help the consumer in such situations.

Are second opinions always valid? Dr. E.G. McCarthy and G.W. Widner reported on a series of cases in the 1974 *New England Journal of Medicine*. They found that 30 percent of patients who voluntarily sought a second opinion were told to avoid surgery. This study reverberated through the halls of the U.S. Congress. It implied that millions of Americans were being subjected to needless surgery.

In 1977 the State of Massachusetts flexed its muscles. It declared that Medicaid recipients must get a second opinion prior to undergoing surgery. Dr. Paul Gertman and associates at the Boston School of Medicine reported their findings in the *New England Journal of Medicine* in May 1980. In this study of 1,591 patients, 180 were advised against surgery.

But there was another twist. These same 180 patients were sent for a third opinion. In 57 cases the second decision was reversed by the consultant. It meant that only 7.7 percent were finally persuaded to avoid surgery.

If I didn't have a medical degree, I hope my guardian angel would nudge me at this point. She'd say, "Don't be followed by the 7.7 percent. Remember the original surgeons knew the patient had to get a second opinion. This makes doctors careful in advising surgery. No doctor can afford to be knife-happy when another surgeon is going to scrutinize his diagnosis. Probably the 30 percent figure is closer to the truth."

When should you see a flashing red light? Let's assume your employer has transferred you to another city. Before the move your family physician had pronounced your health to be good. Now a new physician recommends major abdominal surgery, or he advises your child's tonsils be excised. But you or your child feel fine. You should run, not walk, to another consultant.

Don't forget that some operative procedures have a poor track record. I've mentioned that 300,000 needless hysterectomies are performed every year. Be equally cautious about tonsillectomy, hemorrhoidectomy, gallbladder and varicose vein procedures.

You should also recognize a flashing green light. Don't waste precious time on a second opinion if the diagnosis is cancer, or if you're struck with an attack of acute appendicitis.

Obvious situations will help you separate the necessary from the unnecessary surgery. For instance, suppose you're 45 years of age and develop severe pain in the upper abdomen? X-rays reveal a stone in the gallbladder and the doctor suggests surgery. Most physicians wouldn't advise a delay for a second opinion. Another more severe attack could follow quickly. It's much wiser to have the organ removed during a lull between attacks.

The presence of symptoms also prompts a green light. The 40-year-old woman who suddenly experiences painful periods and heavy, prolonged bleeding has a valid reason for quick action. So does the elderly man who finds it increasingly difficult to urinate.

Remember there are also grey areas when doctors have honest differences of opinion. The conservative surgeon may advise leaving hemorrhoids alone until bleeding and pain become unbearable. Another surgeon may believe in prompt removal for the sake of convenience.

Don't forget there are exceptions to every rule. One of my first patients had no symptoms, but one major complaint. She couldn't go to church any longer. Due to her increasing size, it was impossible for her to get between the pews. The reason? A 33-pound benign ovarian cyst. I didn't suggest a consultation. One look at her abdomen told both of us something was abnormally wrong.

Repeat Caesarean Section or Vaginal Delivery After Caesarean?

Are women's groups right in pressing for this change? Or will some patients get more than they bargained for? Surgeons have always believed, "Once a caesarean always a caesarean." Now feminists are challenging this male-dominated dictum and promoting vaginal delivery after caesarean (VDAC). But their childbearing colleagues are not getting the whole story. It will end in misfortune for some women.

The cry from women, "Once a caesarean, not always a caesarean," is deceptive. If a caesarean is needed in a first pregnancy because the bony pelvis is too small, it will always be needed. But perhaps the patient was unlucky the first time, say female groups. The umbilical cord got caught around the baby's neck, causing a lack of oxygen to the fetus. Or the placenta (afterbirth) prematurely separated from the uterine wall. Why subject these women to another surgical operation when such problems may not recur?

Advocates of VDAC reveal fiercely negative attitudes towards caesarean section. One remarked, "I felt cheated out of a meaningful natural birth. It would have brought me closer to my child." Another mused, "I had the feeling a huge natural force had been abruptly halted."

Today more women are denied the experience of vaginal delivery for very legitimate reasons. Fetal monitors in delivery rooms are detecting fetal distress easier and faster. Breech births, where the baby comes down feet first, are diagnosed more quickly and are delivered with less damage by caesarean. Obstetricians are also opting for less hazardous deliveries because they are wary of medical–legal problems.

I sympathize with them. Natural childbirth has been pushed to unnatural extremes. As architects of their own misfortune, doctors have allowed fathers and sometimes children into the delivery room. What was once a sterile hospital work area now must be equipped with low lights and soft music as if it were an entertainment area. Some hospitals have even introduced checkered tablecloths and a candlelight dinner for the family after the baby is born. In such a Disneyland atmosphere mothers and babies are not expected to suffer and die. If they do, then surely the doctor must have been at fault.

Surgeons had good reason to insist that, "Once a caesarean, always a caesarean." Weakened scar tissue from previous operations sometimes ruptures either before or during labor. This causes massive hemorrhage and fetal death. Today's lower uterine incision results in a stronger scar and less chance of rupture. But pregnant women who have the choice of a repeat caesarean or VDAC should be aware of all the facts.

After years of medical practice I continue to marvel at the perfection of the human body. But there's one area of exception. I remain convinced that the Creator might have devised a better method of childbirth. During labor and delivery the female pelvis sometimes takes an awesome beating. If this is a natural process, then I'd want someone to protect me from it.

Women's advocates never mention the urinary incontinence that plagues some patients after natural childbirth. Some cases require subsequent operations to repair the damaged urinary system. These operations are not always successful. Nor is there any mention of the number of women who undergo hysterectomy following childbirth because supporting ligaments of the uterus have been destroyed by a traumatic delivery. I agree that caesareans have a higher mortality than vaginal deliveries. But to balance the argument, what about the mortality rate of such later corrective operations?

Women's consumer groups would be better advised to unleash an attack elsewhere. On obstetricians who still maintain an unrealistic attitude towards caesareans—the ones who insist on delivering the first child vaginally even if it's a breech, or who advise a 35-year-old woman who has never had a child to have a natural delivery. When needless tragedies occur in such cases, everyone remains silent.

I've often criticized male surgeons for a lingering chauvinism. Some have physically and psychologically mutilated women for years while surgically treating cancer of the breast. They continue to do so even though recent studies prove that the cure rate of breast removal is no better than that of less traumatic procedures. Women have every right to denounce this type of radical surgery.

But can the increased number of Caesareans be blamed totally on male chauvinism? I don't think so. There have been major beneficial advancements in obstetrics. Caesareans are now safer and less traumatic and should be considered an alternate method of childbirth. It's possible that some women get a psychological lift from VDAC, but other patients may get more than they bargained for.

Will You Operate so I Can Play Cards?

Would a reputable surgeon operate just so a patient could play cards? Or is this the best definition of a knife-happy surgeon? The thought crossed my mind as I listened to a patient's complaint. She was 91 and not acutely ill. But for the past year she had been unable to play cards because of urinary stress incontinence. She looked me straight in the eye and insisted that I must cure this annoying problem. But why does this malady affect so many women? And what special traps await business and post-menopausal women?

Stress incontinence and childbirth are irrevocably linked. Today many patients are victims of history. Their children were born in an era when caesarean sections were reserved for only serious life-threatening obstetrical complications. Doctors who performed more than five caesareans in 100 deliveries were considered by colleagues to be practicing poor obstetrics.

Years ago the "art" of obstetrics reigned supreme. Doctors were proud if they could manipulate a large baby through a narrow bony pelvis. I've often seen obstetricians brace their feet against the end of the delivery table and pull with all their strength on forceps around the baby's head. Small wonder some of these children were left with cerebral palsy, and their mothers with urinary incontinence.

Why do some women have difficulty holding their urine? In the normal female abdomen the floor of the bladder lies along the front wall of the vagina. But long arduous labors, large babies, or several pregnancies in rapid succession often cause injury to supporting tissues of the bladder. The result? The bladder may fall down into the vagina, and muscles controlling the urinary opening lose strength. Any increase in abdominal pressure such as laughing or sneezing causes a loss of urine. Even the act of walking or sitting down in a chair can produce an embarrassing situation.

Stress incontinence forces some women into seclusion. They believe they must remain forever social outcasts. Husbands have told me of wives who used to enjoy dancing or were the life of a party. When corrective surgery sometimes failed to relieve the horrendous problem, they refused to go anywhere. The more cases I see of stress incontinence, the more I'm convinced that prevention is better than cure.

How will future career women be affected by this chronic annoyance? For some businesswomen there's good news. Doctors now have a more realistic attitude towards caesarean sections. This, along with the tendency to smaller families, will help prevent stress incontinence. But there are still special pitfalls for professional women.

Today many working women are postponing pregnancy. When they do, they forget one vital fact. Women in their 30s are like aging baseball players. They're more likely to strike out. Some mature women can't get pregnant. Others will develop pregnancy complications. Still others, because of difficult labors and less pliable tissues, will end up with stress incontinence.

Does this mean I'd advocate caesareans for all mature career women? No. But women should take another look at the pros and cons of this operation. It should no longer be considered the route of last resort. Rather, it can be a sound, alternate choice for delivery.

Career women often fall into this error. At 35 years of age they realize they may only have one pregnancy. Today they are also subjected to an abundance of opinion about the joys of natural childbirth. Many will opt for an emotional experience without realizing the possible anatomical consequences.

Post-menopausal women make another mistake. Few women get through natural delivery scot-free. The majority escape stress incontinence. But some relaxation of the vaginal wall always occurs. Aging causes further deterioration of tissue supporting the bladder. This weakness is accentuated when there is also a lack of the female hormone, estrogen. Yet, because of scare tactics linking estrogen to cancer, many women fail to use this useful hormone. A more realistic use of estrogen would help prevent many cases of incontinence.

What about my 91-year-old patient who wanted to play cards? N.R. Crump, former president of Canadian Pacific Railway, once gave some apocryphal advice about catching porcupines. "Sneak up and slam a washtub over him," said Crump. "This gives you a place to sit and think about what you're going to do with him." This approach also pays dividends when you're weighing the pros and cons of surgery on the aged. So I used it.

But biological age was the ultimate clue in this case. The patient was young in spirit and health. Now she's back playing cards. I'll bet she's also picking up all the money.

Revolutionary Cure for Urinary Incontinence

Thousands of healthy women suffer from urinary incontinence, but a new technique now will relieve the majority of them of this embarrassing annoyance. This surgery differs from operations used in the past, but it should become a routine procedure to treat urinary stress incontinence.

Stress incontinence occurs not only as a result of childbirth. Some women are born with weak vaginal tissues that break down with the passing years. Such patients eventually begin to feel a "bearing down" sensation in the vagina or notice a mass at the vaginal entrance.

But the loss of urine that so often accompanies a fallen bladder is the major problem. Women with this trouble begin to feel like social outcasts. Some even go into seclusion rather than face discomfiting situations.

Relieving women of this bothersome complaint has always been difficult. The time-honored technique involved stitching the prolapsed tissues back into their normal position. But this is easier said than done. These tissues are often extremely thin. Or severely damaged by childbirth. All too often it's like trying to stitch blotting paper together. Initial results might seem promising, but in a few months the damaged tissues sometimes pull apart and urine loss returns. To prevent this complication someone had to invent a better mousetrap.

The Department of Gynecology at Toronto Western Hospital has been developing an imaginative approach for several years. Like understanding the advantages of the round wheel over the square one, it's amazing that it's taken so long for surgeons to see the merits of this technique.

Researchers at Toronto Western knew that a synthetic material called merseline mesh was being used to repair abdominal hernias. They decided to utilize this mesh to provide extra support to fallen vaginal tissues. But there was one problem. Surgeons repairing a hernial defect in the abdomen can always find strong tissues nearby to hold the mesh in place. Such tissues are non-existent in the vagina. There's no point in suturing a piece of merseline mesh to a weak support. The weakest link fails and the incontinence returns.

The surgeons eventually found an innovative way to provide firm support for the opening of the bladder. They created small tunnels alongside of the pubic bones and tucked the mesh into these indentations. In this way the merseline mesh sling could be suspended snugly underneath the bladder opening. The majority of patients with this problem have achieved lasting results when this technique was used.

Initially there was some fear that this foreign material would be rejected by the body. But in a series of over 300 cases this has rarely happened. Now we know that merseline mesh is well accepted by the vaginal tissues.

The majority of patients have little trouble after surgery. A catheter routinely drains the bladder for five days. Once it's removed, most patients are able to void normally. But placing a merseline sling under the bladder does cause more swelling than the standard operation. Therefore a few patients need a catheter reinserted until the edema subsides. This may add a few more days to the hospital convalescence. It's a small price to pay for a final, lasting result.

I see an increasing need for this operation in the years ahead. Many working women are postponing pregnancy until their 30s. They also want to experience the joys of natural childbirth. But some of these women will have more difficult labors due to the less pliable vaginal tissues. This will leave more women with urinary stress incontinence.

We also have an aging population. Vaginal tissues, like other parts of the human body, begin to sag in the elderly. This is particularly true if estrogen isn't taken to help keep the vaginal tissues thick and healthy.

What is my personal opinion of this surgery? Common sense tells me that researchers at Toronto Western Hospital have created a whole new dimension in pelvic surgery. As a gynecologist who has had to cope with many difficult cases of stress incontinence over the years, I now enthusiastically use this technique on patients. The results confirm that the merseline mesh sling is superior. I hope that more pelvic surgeons make use of it in the future.

But what about the countless women who have already undergone one or more operations in the attempt to cure this trouble? A woman from Vancouver writes, "I have to use hand towels and a plastic covering at night for protection. Even a short walk to the store is fraught with the possibility of embarrassment. I can no longer visit friends' homes. After two operations I'm afraid of doctors and hospitals. But I'm desperate for a cure."

Another woman from California says, "I have to use a stop-watch to remind me it's time to go to the bathroom. But I still can't keep dry. Anyone with this annoyance can forget about glamorous clothes."

For one poor woman, the problem caused an orthopedic injury. She says, "In my rush to get to the bathroom I fell off the toilet and injured my hip. Thank God someone is trying to help us. It would be a joy to be able to go on a trip and enjoy the few years I have left."

Some patients were angered at having been given false hopes by the doctor. They were assured that either vaginal or abdominal surgery would cure them and last a lifetime. But after the third or fourth operation they had become convinced theirs was a hopeless condition. All of these patients asked whether the merseline mesh sling could help them.

The answer is no. This vaginal procedure is performed only on women who have never had previous surgery to solve this annoyance. But after one failed operation, different surgical approaches must be carried out. Some patients can be cured by an abdominal operation. If this has already been attempted, Toronto Western Hospital employs a two-team attack.

One surgeon working vaginally frees up the scarred vaginal tissues and places a strip of synthetic marlex material underneath the weakened bladder. He than makes two small tunnels alongside the pubic bones and pushes the ends of the marlex strip upwards into the abdominal cavity.

A second surgeon has already made an abdominal incision and catches hold of the ends of the marlex strip. These ends are then stitched to strong ligaments. The weakened bladder is now positioned like a person sitting on the seat of a swing, with the ends of the rope attached to the limbs of a strong tree.

Does it work? Regrettably, the old adage still applies. Two things are certain in life, death and taxes. The best results are obtained when patients have had one failed vaginal operation followed by unsuccessful abdominal surgery. But even after three or four ineffectual operations the two-team approach can and often does relieve women of urinary incontinence.

There are some general guidelines. First of all, remember that some women with urinary incontinence do not have injured bladders. Rather, the bladder may not be functioning properly for other reasons. Surgery will not correct these cases. To separate those patients who will be aided by this operation from cases of bladder malfunction, urodynamic studies must be undertaken.

But let's assume you require additional surgery after one or more failed operations. Remember that a weakened, injured bladder reacts like an enraged, wounded tiger. It is complex and supersensitive. No one would ever ask an inexperienced hunter to track down and kill this animal. Similarly, it requires a team of super-specialists to handle this tricky organ. The best place to find such surgeons is in a university hospital. Your family doctor can be helpful in guiding you to the best care.

14

Sex

One column of mine provoked more reader response than just about any other. Here it is reprinted in its entirety:

Should we ever laugh at disease? I never thought so. But recently I came across a study of a rare disease and couldn't stop chuckling. Hopefully this column will prevent someone from becoming case number 68. And perhaps, for a change, women will have a good laugh about men.

When patient X was admitted to the hospital emergency department at 1:00 a.m. he was in obvious trouble. But the examining doctors were puzzled. They were unable to make an immediate diagnosis.

The patient was pale, nervous, and agitated. His skin was cold and clammy. Assuming he was in shock, physicians made a thorough examination for blood loss. They were surprised at what they found. The man's penis was markedly swollen, measuring seven inches in diameter. The patient was transferred to the operating room for removal of a massive blood clot.

How had such an injury occurred? The man was reluctant to explain at first. But the story was eventually revealed. He had been masturbating vigorously, when he heard a sudden snap. Pain and swelling of the penis followed.

The diagnosis was a fractured penis. This became the sixty-seventh case to be reported in world medical journals. Further reading of the other 66 cases provided more laughs. Especially entertaining were the causes of the fractured penis syndrome.

T.L. Arnold reported several cases in the 1977 *Journal of Urology*. He concluded that the injury occurs only when the penis is erect. The most common cause was a direct blow to the penis or bending it.

Some males suffered the embarrassing malady after bumping into a chair or bedpost during the night. Others were kicked during a fight. One man's penis was smashed during the attack of an animal.

Other scenarios require a vivid imagination. They prove that making love may be hazardous to your health. For example, one Romeo was injured while having intercourse in a moving car. He was thrown against the dashboard when the car came to a sudden stop. Another occurred when the erect penis struck the saddle knob of a motorcycle. One patient slammed his penis in a car door. That takes considerable skill and planning.

It appears that lying down to make love is the safest position. Doctors reported a patient suffered injury while having intercourse in a standing position. He must have been quite a lover. His partner suddenly fainted and her fall fractured his penis.

Dr. Ashraf is a urologist at Penderfields General Hospital in Wakefield, England. He reported several other cases in the 1978 *Journal of Urology*. One of his patients was an 18-year-old shepherd. He was sitting in a tree watching sheep. But he fell asleep and landed on a wooden bar. When he fell, his penis was erect and was fractured.

A 26-year-old man's honeymoon was suddenly ended. His penis slipped during intercourse, striking his wife's hard pubic bone. There was a clicking sound and the penis was bent. The man refused to go to hospital. Six weeks later he returned to his physician with a slightly bent penis. Another newlywed fractured his while rolling over in the bed during an erection.

How is the penis fractured? The tissues of the male organ are surrounded by a tough fibrous sheath called the tunica albuginea. This becomes thinner during erection. Severe strain or a sudden blow can tear it, causing a snapping sound. Previous urinary infections may also predispose the tissue to this problem.

Treatment depends on the severity of the injury. The majority require pressure dressings, ice packs, and anti-inflammatory drugs to decrease the swelling. Tranquilizers are also given to calm the patient and to avoid further erections for several days. A foley catheter is frequently needed to enable the patient to void. And some urologists have used tongue depressors as a form of splint.

Surgery is performed when there is a massive blood clot present. Or when the urinary tube is also torn. Most patients are discharged in two weeks and normal sexual activity can be resumed in about eight weeks. A few males are left with a slightly bent penis.

Some of these unfortunate victims suffered depression following injury. Psychiatric care eased the short-term trauma. But one patient committed suicide a year later.

Men have been known to laugh at some of the embarrassing medical problems of women. Now females can have the last laugh. Is anyone anxious to be case number 68?

The Case of the Amorous Nurse

How could a compassionate nurse do this to a doctor? I could reach only one conclusion. She was either mean or very amorous. As we've seen, above, men already face hair-raising problems from some sexual encounters with the so-called "weaker sex." Now a medical report from Finland alerts males to another hazard of lovemaking. It's just a matter of time until it occurs in North America. Who will be number one?

The doctor involved in this case was the victim. But he put off seeking medical attention. Four weeks after a sexual encounter there was no doubt that something was dramatically wrong. He couldn't raise his left shoulder. The trapezius, the shoulder's main muscle, was tender, and he had difficulty lifting his left arm.

Twelve weeks later the situation had not improved. The shoulder was still painful. Occasionally the left arm had to be supported to relieve the aching muscle. Carrying objects became a major problem. Jogging and swimming merely aggravated the pain in the shoulder because of the weakened condition of the trapezius muscle.

Six months later without treatment the ache had almost vanished. The shoulder had recovered most of its former strength. And the muscle atrophy was no longer present.

What had happened to this healthy 28-year-old male physician? He gave no history of suffering in the past with either muscle or nervous disease. But late one night he had dated a sympathetic nurse. During the heat of lovemaking, she bit him in the neck.

Inadvertently the front edge of the trapezius muscle was damaged in the encounter. It was described later by the physician as "a rather vigorous bite," even though the skin was not torn by his ardent partner's teeth. Immediately following the bite, his shoulder was paralyzed. And soon a dull ache spread from shoulder to the upper arm. The lovemaking ended abruptly because of the paralysis and pain.

This doctor had evidently been a good student of anatomy. He made his own diagnosis of accessory nerve palsy. Knowing that this nerve lies in a very superficial location in the neck, he was aware that it was vulnerable to injury.

Why do people bite during lovemaking? In the process of evolution we've lost our hairy tails, but we haven't thrown away the animal habit of biting. C.S. Ford and F.A. Beach in *Patterns of Sexual Behavior* give ample evidence of biting in the animal world. The males of many lower mammals often grasp the neck of the female to control her during mating.

Studies by anthropologists show that who bites whom varies in different societies. For example, some human cultures admit to biting and pulling hair during lovemaking. In such societies both sexes show affection that way. But a study of the Trobriand Islanders revealed that it's only the women who inflict significant injuries this way.

What about North America? It's not earthshaking news that the accessory trapezius nerve can be injured. We've known for years that it can be damaged occasionally during surgical procedures on the thyroid gland. Or when a doctor is removing a malignant tumor from this location. Other cases of accessory nerve palsy are the result of war injuries.

Dr. A. Norden describes another hazard in a Scandinavian medical journal. A man accidentally walked into a ladder while carrying a wooden beam on his shoulder. The beam struck his neck, resulting in temporary paralysis. And Dr. D.S. Bell, writing in the *British Medical Journal*, detailed another case. His patient tried unsuccessfully to hang himself. He only injured the shoulder muscle.

But the report on "Biting Palsy of the Accessory Nerve" published in the April 1980 issue of the *Journal of Neurology, Neurosurgery and Psychiatry* is a unique case. I couldn't find any other cases in medical literature.

Who will be number one in North America? It won't be me. Researching these sexual hazards has made me a nervous wreck. Now I'm even afraid to shake hands.

But there will be a number one. Recently I asked a teenage patient about a severe bruise on her neck. She explained it was "a hickey." I'm sure she also thought, "You dum dum. Haven't you ever seen a love-bite before?"

The Dilemma of Teenage Sex

Mrs. H.N. of Windsor writes, "My daughter says that most of her high-school friends are no longer virgins. Recently one of them became pregnant. Would you do a column on teenage sex and how parents can cope with this matter?"

Many letters are sent to me about sexual problems of all kinds. A large percentage come from concerned parents who find themselves on the horns of a dilemma. They don't want to appear too prudish and old-fashioned and yet are deeply concerned that their sons or daughters are playing a hazardous game. They ask over and over again, "How can we handle this problem?"

Today we live in a liberalized sexual society. On the surface one would think that modern teenagers, would be the most knowledgeable generation ever. But this is not the case. Many young people have simply jumped out of the Victorian frying pan into a blazing fire. The burns may be deep and long lasting.

An increasing number of teenagers are asking for the birth control pill in their headlong rush into sexual freedom. However, in their desire to escape from unwanted pregnancies, they have wandered into areas where they are babes in the woods. Their male counterparts also have discovered that there's more to sex than pregnancy.

Teenagers are not tuned in to dangers of a free-wheeling sexual relationship. Like their parents, they believe that getting venereal disease means contracting gonorrhea or syphilis. Yet, several common problems such as trichomonas, fungus, and bacterial infections are also easily transmitted by sexual contact. They won't shorten a teenager's life, but they can be extremely irritating and tedious to eradicate.

It's a tragedy to see a 14-year-old girl develop these annoying diseases from premature sexual activity. It is an utter catastrophe when she contracts one or both of the big venereal diseases while jumping from one amorous affair to another. Moreover, these diseases are not always diagnosed early because the symptoms may be minimal. This sets the stage for long-term problems.

For teenage youths, an undiagnosed gonorrheal infection may result in troublesome prostatitis that goes on for years. For teenage girls, this infection can produce sterility and chronic pelvic symptoms. And for both sexes an untreated case of syphilis can have disastrous results in later life. Doing your own thing with sex isn't all roses and honey.

How can parents help children to circumvent these problems? First of all, they have to rid themselves of some major misconceptions about sex education. Some think that the less their children know the better. Others assume that they will learn about sex soon enough from their friends. Eventually all children pick up the facts from a variety of sources. Yet what they assimilate is often distorted and clothed in such vulgarity that it leads to lifetime fallacies about sex.

Too many parents have the wrong idea about sex education in the schools. They believe that emphasis on birth control automatically leads to sexual promiscuity. It's like saying that the more you know about sex the more you'll want to try it out. Or that ignorance is a good thing in sex or anything else.

This year a large number of Toronto's secondary schools refused to participate in Birth Control Week. Some principals admitted they were afraid of parental reaction to sex education. And while the VD rate was escalating and thousands of needless teenage abortions were being done, some health officials were still debating whether this instruction should be called birth control or family planning. No wonder teenagers go down the wrong road when parents argue over such trivia.

Parents should support and demand sex education in the schools, because most of them are poorly equipped to handle it in the home. Some are too embarrassed to discuss the subject. Others are so preoccupied with their own sexual troubles that they impart the wrong information.

Crude, clumsy attempts at teaching sex may be worse than none at all. The disapproving frown, embarrassed silences, or the innuendo that sex is dirty or evil won't wipe out teenage problems or prepare them for a healthy attitude towards sex.

Parents also make the mistake of putting off explanations. Many girls are therefore shocked at the first sight of menstruation. Similarly, a boy's first ejaculation can be a frightening experience if it occurs during a dream or masturbation, if no one has told him about it.

Fewer teenagers will fall into pitfalls if the techniques of sex, birth control, and the hazards of VD are mandatory subjects in our schools. But parents can't leave everything to the teachers. Good living starts in the home, and too often children emulate their parents' poor behavior. Adults who jump from one marriage to another or who stagger from tavern to tavern can hardly expect good conduct from teenagers.

A research group once called homes in the evening to see how many parents knew the whereabouts of their children. To their surprise the telephone was most often answered by teenagers who didn't know where to find their parents. That's a poor way for adults to the play the game.

Students Should Pack Porcupine Caution into Their Traveling Bags

Veterinarians tell me that porcupines make love very, very carefully. I can believe it. But will North American students traveling to other countries this summer show similar restraint? How many will return home with serious complications from sexually transmitted disease? Many of these tragedies can be prevented. But they'll need double-barreled sexual protection to accomplish it.

Students reading this column will turn cynical at this point. They'll say, "Gifford-Jones, you're just like our parents. You're going to use scare tactics and lecture us on sexual abstinence. But times have changed and you should know it."

Indeed, times have changed. I see it every day in my office. And I know it's impossible to change sexual standards with an 800-word sermon. Preaching is not my business. But the cold, unemotional medical facts of sexual behavior do concern me. Especially ways to keep venereal disease statistics from climbing.

Students will forget one fact this summer. Sex and science are still miles apart. A jumbo jet and computerized technology will carry them quickly to all parts of the world, but modern science still hasn't discovered a jumbo jet way to prevent VD. Medical science can transplant hearts and cure many problems that previously killed people. There are also better ways to treat syphilis and gonorrhea. But the best defence against these problems is still prevention.

Here's another fact. World health figures show that sexually transmitted disease is escalating in most countries. A few years ago, Dr. Thornstein Guthe, former chief medical officer of the World Health Organization, aptly summed up the situation. He told a scientific meeting in Warsaw that, "There is now a common market in venereal disease."

That's why young people who board a 747 jet have to think about double-barreled sexual protection. The birth control pill has been a great boon in many ways. It has liberated women, and men, from the fear of pregnancy. But this contraceptive and the IUD have exposed both to the greater hazards of VD.

So here's the next important fact. The condom is the only contraceptive that provides double protection, from pregnancy and VD. Casanova, the great lover, thought it was a safe approach. Things haven't changed since his time.

Students might decide at this point to go on the offensive. They may say, "That may be good advice for some people. But it doesn't apply to me. I'm not the type to wander into the back alleys of Hamburg, Istanbul, or Singapore. I may indulge in sex. But I'll be careful to pick the right partner."

Facts show that this is still a risky move. VD is no longer the sole preserve of prostitutes or women of the streets. The questionable distinction of the prostitute as the main source of infection has been replaced by the availability of the casual pick-up. The most sophisticated and fastidious young people become afflicted with venereal disease after a momentary indiscretion. After taking precautions against pregnancy, they are horrified to find themselves in another bind.

Don't forget another fact. The germs that cause venereal disease are getting stronger in some parts of the world. One recent medical report referred to a new resistant strain of gonorrhea as "King Clap." It's a virulent type with a lot of muscle that laughs at penicillin.

So whatever way you slice the cake one fact stands out. The best defence is the first defence. Condoms are not 100 percent foolproof against VD, but if used correctly they can eradicate much of the trouble. Students need not return home with pelvic infection and possible lifelong sterility. Others need not suffer recurring attacks of prostatitis and other problems.

I hope students will keep the porcupine in mind when they step off the jumbo jet this summer. It could help to prevent many tragic cases of syphilis and gonorrhea.

Unfortunately that's not the whole story. Most people haven't heard that there are other sexually transmitted diseases. Some may not want to hear about them. But this isn't a conspiracy to preclude enjoyment of travel abroad. It's merely providing you with plain, simple facts.

Why is everyone so badly informed about these common diseases? One reason is they're not always due to sexual intercourse. For instance, females may develop a vaginal fungus infection when antibiotics are prescribed for a boil or sore throat. Women can pick up trichomonas from the neighborhood swimming pool. But in most cases it's impossible to pinpoint accurately the source of the problem. Doctors can only make a calculated guess.

Yet one point is beyond dispute. Sexual intercourse does play a major role in spreading these diseases. And due to increased sexual freedom, sexually transmitted disease (STD) has become epidemic in North America and elsewhere.

STD makes syphilis and gonorrhea look like poor cousins. Some reports say there are a million cases a year in Canada. Exact figures are impossible to obtain, but there's a simple way to determine the extent of the problem. Daily in my office, I see two or three cases.

Trichomonas is the most common sexually transmitted disease. It's a small, single-celled protozoan organism. Males who contact this infection are usually unaware of its presence. But females normally complain of an irritating vaginal discharge and odor.

Monilia is another common STD. It's a fungus infection that adheres to the vaginal walls and looks like cottage cheese. This problem causes intense itching. Several kinds of bacterial infection are also transmitted by sexual contact.

Is STD a serious problem? Both trichomonas and monilia are not life-threatening diseases. But they can certainly decrease the pleasures of singing in a Munich beer hall or enjoying a full moon over Naples Bay. Treatment usually results in speedy relief of symptoms. But resistant cases that fail to respond to a variety of drugs are not rare. Some people have recurring attacks that last for months or years.

Less fortunate students may return home with extremely difficult and trying problems. Herpes genitales, a virus infection, produces small, fluid-filled vesicles around the genital organs. They form several days after exposure and eventually break, leaving painful, ulcerated areas. The sores gradually heal and may never recur. But about half the cases return in six months. Some students suffer repeated attacks, since there's no known cure.

Other infections, such as chlamydia, causes inflammation of the eyes. The disease can also involve the rectum, urinary tube, and genital organs. All told there are about 20 of these non-traditional venereal diseases.

Males are also more prone to develop a condition called "non-specific urethritis." It's an inflammation of the urinary tube which can spread to the prostate gland. Patients complain of discharge, painful urination, and a gnawing pain deep in the rectal area.

What is the primary message for this summer's young travelers? Students must realize that being on the move automatically places them in a high-risk category. Moreover, reports stress that 60 percent of STD occurs in persons under 24 years of age.

Of course, most sexual contact does not result in syphilis or gonorrhea. Lady Luck is sometimes on your side. But for the sexually active, trichomonas and other types of STD are difficult to avoid. They're simply too prevalent in this free-wheeling society today.

André Gide, the novelist and philosopher, once started a lecture by emphasizing, "All this has been said before, but since nobody listened, it must be said again." That's why I want to repeat something I've stressed before. VD is no longer just associated with prostitutes and women of the streets. The main source of infection is now the casual contact. And STD crosses all social boundaries.

So in this roaring jet age, students still have only one choice if they intend to indulge in sex. The condom remains the only preventative against VD. Without this protection students are virtually assured of contact with STD.

If you want to gamble, spend a day at Monte Carlo and get it out of your system. But don't gamble with STD. The dice are loaded and you may ruin an enjoyable trip. Bon voyage.

Washroom Posters, Inc.

Some readers may think I've developed an abnormal attraction to public washrooms. I've questioned whether women should sit on public toilet seats. Now I'm invading that private sanctuary again—to hang posters on their walls.

Research shows that washrooms are prime locations for teaching teenagers about "Me Tarzan, you Jane."

Washroom walls have always been used to pass along comments. They're seldom the right kind. But like roadside signs, it's hard to avoid reading them. For years we've been missing the boat. It's time to put washroom walls to more productive use.

Dr. Alan Grogono is an associate professor of anesthesiology at the New York Upstate Medical Center. He suggested putting washroom walls to use when he was a medical student in England. But for a different purpose.

Professor Grogono outlined his theory during a recent medical conference. In England midwives are used for routine obstetrical deliveries. They're trained to be efficient in testing the urine of pregnant women for sugar. Student midwives are also required to check their own urine once a year as a precautionary measure. But they were continually negligent about bringing in samples.

Dr. Grogono suggested a notice be placed in the women's washroom requiring a urine sample before the first lecture. The response was almost 100 percent. The desk of the head nurse was promptly covered with urine bottles.

This success triggered another interesting experiment. Student midwives are also taught the technique of cardio-pulmonary resuscitation (CPR). Dr. Grogono decided to transfer 25 of the most pertinent facts about CPR onto posters. He placed them in one washroom for three weeks. But he purposely left the posters out of another dormitory washroom.

Three weeks later the students were given an examination. They were asked to answer questions selected from the American Heart Association's basic life support test. Students from the dormitory where posters had been placed got the highest grades. Their score was even better than those who had already been certified in CPR.

Dr. Grogono's idea may be the way to teach sex education to teenagers. Present tactics aren't working. Every year an increasing number of teenagers have pregnancies and abortions. For example, the Alberta Medical Association warned that teenage abortion is escalating at the rate of 16 percent a year. The number of repeat abortions is climbing by almost 20 percent a year.

What would we do if measles, polio, or Legionnaires Disease was increasing at that rate? A public outcry would be heard from coast to coast. The government would appoint a special task force to investigate. We'd spend millions of dollars to find a cure. But we don't need expensive commissions to pinpoint the reasons for teenage pregnancies.

Illustrating washroom posters is not my specialty. But after talking to dozens of pregnant teenagers every year, I know what needs to be said. The largest posters should hammer home one point: If teenage girls assume pregnancy won't happen, it will. We need to stress the disastrous effect of this common assumption.

A poster of an old Tarzan movie would fill the bill. The one in which he says, "Me Tarzan, you Jane." We could persuade an updated Tarzan to add,

"You, Jane, go on pill. No want little Tarzans swinging from vines." And Jane might retort in a huff, "You, Tarzan, use condom?"

Teenagers could speculate on another poster. What direction would Tarzan swing if Jane became pregnant? Would he still play the good guy role? Or would he act like so many other males and grab the swiftest vine to Bulla Bulla land? Would he announce that it wasn't his fault? That she must have wandered off in the bush with someone else? That he'd been sterilized by a witch doctor? Or that he just didn't give a damn? It was her problem and she would have to fend for herself.

An enterprising entrepreneur might start Washroom Posters Inc. Tarzan could appear in the washrooms of both sexes. His macho image might be more effective in teaching birth control, even good hygiene and physical fitness.

Washroom Posters Inc. would be a financial bonanza. There's a captive audience. Space could be sold to companies for constructive messages. And the Tarzan lessons might sink into young brains. It's worth a try.

The Herpes Epidemic

Some days I feel so totally helpless that I may as well be a witch doctor. This sensation overtakes me every time I make a diagnosis of herpes simplex type 2. There's still no help in sight for the patient with this invisible, incurable virus. And without even realizing the risk, millions of young people are in contact with this dread disease. Why has this problem reached epidemic proportions? And is there any way to prevent this infection?

Researchers have labeled this "the virus of love" or "the new sexual leprosy." But history shows it's not a new problem. Blisters associated with fever were recognized more than 2,000 years ago. And the Roman emperor Tiberius tried to eradicate herpes by banning kissing.

Herpes simplex belongs to a family of more than 70 viruses. But only a few cause human diseases such as chicken pox, shingles, infectious mononucleosis, and birth defects. The ones causing venereal disease are herpes 1 and 2. Type 1 produces cold sores around the mouth. It can also cause eye ailments that if untreated may lead to blindness. Type 2 occurs around the genital area and sometimes on thighs and buttocks.

This virus has recently gone on a rampage. It started with the sexual revolution of the 1960s and proves that free-wheeling sex in the 1980s carries with it overwhelming liabilities.

Dr. Paul Wiesner, director of the venereal disease division at Atlanta's Centers for Disease Control, has some grim figures. He estimates that about 30 percent of the sexually active population have been exposed to this virus. Other authorities say that 1 in 200 patients attending gynecological clinics has herpes, and that 1 in every 100 pregnant women carries the virus.

This year half a million North Americans will develop telltale symptoms. About two to eight days after contact with the virus, small, itchy, red bumps will appear in the genital area. They're usually so close that they join together. Two to three days after their appearance they rupture, producing shallow, painful ulcers. And when the vesicles break they release millions of infectious particles.

Victims get a false sense of security when the sores heal in about 10 days. But the virus doesn't leave the body. Instead it goes into hiding in the nerves near the lower spinal cord. They remain in that location for the rest of the person's life.

How often the virus returns varies from patient to patient. Some women complain of painful lesions during each menstrual period. Others suffer recurrences under severe stress or if there's a sudden change in temperature. But there is no way to predict if the virus will strike again in weeks, months, or years.

Doctors have noticed another trend in patients who contact sexually transmitted diseases. These people often have more than one infection. For example, in one series 90 percent of the patients with herpes also had gonorrhea; 40 percent had a fungus infection; 25 percent suffered from trichomonas; and 12 percent had venereal warts.

The long-term consequences can be catastrophic for pregnant women. Eighty percent of the babies who pass through an infected canal catch this disease. And of these, 50 percent will either die or develop severe neurological complications. For this reason women with active herpes are delivered by caesarean section.

Herpes 1 has also been associated with the development of cancer of the cervix. It's still debatable whether this virus is responsible for the 18,000 cases that occur in the U.S. and Canada every year. But it's especially important that women with herpes have regular pelvic examinations. The Pap smear can detect malignant changes in the cells years before they become outright cancers. This test can often diagnose herpes. Unfortunately doctors don't yet have a miracle drug to cure the infection.

How can young people escape herpes? They must first realize that the birth control pill is a double-edged sword. By removing the fear of pregnancy it's created an epidemic of herpes and other venereal diseases. More young people should re-examine the virtues of old-fashioned morality. Those who cast it aside should at least return to the use of condoms. This would help to fight herpes infections. It would also decrease the times that I feel no better than a witch doctor.

Most Frequent Questions About Herpes

How Do You Know that Genital Herpes Is Present?
The diagnosis of herpes is pinpointed 95 percent of the time by a typical course of symptoms. About 2 to 10 days after the virus enters the body red bumps appear which quickly become itchy, painful, fluid-filled blisters. A few days later the blisters rupture and become ulcers, gradually form scabs, and heal in

two to three weeks. If they keep recurring in the same place the diagnosis of herpes simplex is even more certain. The sores are usually accompanied by fever, headache, pain in the muscles, and a general malaise.

Can a Blood Test Diagnose Herpes?
A blood test is of limited value. A positive test merely indicates that the person was infected with the virus at some time. This may have occurred many years ago and the patient has never had another attack.

What Is the Best Way to Diagnose Herpes?
A culture provides the ultimate answer. Doctors take a specimen from the lesions and place it in a culture consisting of living cells that are maintained at body temperature. If the virus grows in this medium the sores are due to herpes.

Do You Need a Break in the Skin to Contract Herpes?
No. The mucous membrane around the genital area and the skin are both porous enough to allow the virus to enter.

Can Two People Who Have Herpes Reinfect Each Other?
Herpes does not confer total immunity. It's therefore possible to get more of the same virus if patients fail to practice prevention during an attack. Some authorities say that the introduction of additional viruses increases the chance of recurrence. Other experts believe that the extra viruses have no effect on the number of attacks. But plain horse sense indicates it's wise to forgo sex while lesions are present. Or when you believe an attack is starting. We know that the herpes virus is present during the early symptoms of an attack.

How Many Attacks of Herpes Will I Have to Endure?
It's impossible to give an exact answer to this question. But there is some good news. Many patients never develop the recurrent form of the disease. The number of people who suffer just one attack is not known. Some authorities say it's as high as 50 percent. Other patients see reactivation of the virus so infrequently the recurrences are of little consequence. It's believed that only 25 to 40 percent of North Americans have frequent attacks.

How Often Will the Attacks Strike?
This varies from person to person. The virus may occur just once every few years. But it can also occur with uncanny regularity, monthly, twice a month, or many times a year. Some patients may have attacks every month, then have relief for long intervals.

What Should I Do When the Sores Are Present?
Cold compresses, painting the lesions with betadine, an iodine solution, and infra-red light may decrease the pain and itching. Keep the area clean and dry and avoid scratching and rubbing the sores. This will help to prevent secondary bacterial infection and the transfer of the virus to other parts of the body. Wash hands often, and never touch the sores and then rub your eyes. And don't expose others to the infection by indulging in sexual activity.

Does Herpes Cause Cancer?
We know that the herpes virus can transform normal cells into defective ones.

Studies also confirm that cancer of the cervix is many times more common in women with genital herpes than among women without this disease. But there is no conclusive proof that herpes actually causes female malignancy. Prudence dictates, however, that women with herpes should have regular Pap smears to detect any early changes which may lead to cancer.

Is Genital Herpes a Serious Disease?

Compared to other sexually transmitted diseases the answer is no. For instance, gonorrhea can result in sterility. Untreated syphilis can cause insanity, blindness, paralysis, and death from vascular complications. Herpes is usually more annoying than dangerous. The only exceptions are when herpes is transmitted to either the eye or the brain.

How Can I Avoid the Complications of Herpes?

Can herpes cause serious life-threatening problems? The answer is usually no. For the great majority of patients with either genital or oral herpes, it is simply a bothersome annoyance. But you should be aware of two exceptions to the rule. Herpes keratitis is one of the leading causes of blindness in North America. And herpes encephalitis of the brain also causes death in some cases. Why do these complications occur? And how can some of them be prevented?

Doctors disagree on the number of cases of herpes keratitis that occur every year. The National Institute of Health in the U.S. in 1979 estimated that 500,000 cases occurred annually. Other prominent eye specialists say it's somewhere between 50,000 and 100,000.

Patients often cause their own problems by "autoinoculation"—in other words, the simple touch of an active herpes lesion can transfer the infection to the eye when the eye is rubbed inadvertently. This can also happen when patients with herpes of the lip use their own saliva to moisten contact lenses prior to insertion.

In addition to self-transfer the virus can enter the eye by a biological accident. During the phase when the herpes virus is inactive it remains in a nerve cluster called the trigeminal ganglia. When it eventually comes out of hibernation, it travels along the nerve pathways to the lips. On very rare occasions a virus may get sidetracked and migrate along the nerves leading to the eye. There is no way that patients can prevent this from happening.

Symptoms are the same whether the virus enters the eye from autoinoculation or by a biological accident. Patients complain initially of an irritated feeling as if something was in the eye. Later on there is pain, an increased sensitivity to light and herpetic lesions may appear on the surface of the eye. Sometimes the viral lesions remain confined to the outer part of the eye, but the virus may penetrate into deeper structures.

During this phase of the infection, the human body's immune system starts to fight the virus and eventually gets the upper hand. But by this time damage to the eye may be so extensive that vision is either partially or totally destroyed. And eye examination by a physician shows that the normally transparent cornea has been marred by scar tissue. Luckily, in mild cases, the infection is limited to the conjunctiva, thus sparing the cornea. Some cases may also be resolved spontaneously, causing little or no damage.

Once herpes attacks the eye it can recur just as in other parts of the body. Dr. Deborah Pavav-Langston, a professor of ophthalmology at the Harvard Medical School, estimates that ocular herpes recurs in 50 percent of cases:

Herpes encephalitis is an extremely rare complication. Some authorities contend that no more than 100 cases occur annually. Others place the number at about 4,000 in North America every year. Unlike ocular herpes, encephalitis cannot be caused by genital herpes. It is associated exclusively with oral herpes and is always due to a biological accident. Why the virus chooses the nerve passageways to the brain is unknown.

The onset of encephalitis is associated with headache, fever, muscle pain, weakness, speech problems, and personality changes. Normally the patient's condition deteriorates, seizures occur, and finally coma. The infection is fatal in about 70 percent of cases. Those who survive are usually left with permanent brain damage. Unlike cells in other parts of the body, once brain cells are destroyed or damaged they cannot be replaced. A few patients are lucky—the infection is mild and the part of the brain affected does not leave the patient with major disability.

Antiviral agents are now available to treat ocular herpes, but they must be used quickly before damage occurs to the eye. The drugs unfortunately are not cures. The treatment must be repeated each time there is a recurrence.

Drugs are also available to cure encephalitis, but the timing of administration is crucial. Diagnosis, however, is difficult to make in the early stages. Patients and doctors often mistake early symptoms for a minor illness such as flu. Regrettably the encephalitis virus usually wins the race against time, and patients are left with varying degrees of brain damage.

Patients with recurrent attacks of herpes cannot prevent these biological accidents. But some cases of ocular herpes can be prevented by taking care to wash hands frequently when active lesions are present. And remembering never to rub the eyes.

Treatment of Herpes

Knowing what not to do in this case is just as important as rushing off in all directions to do something. Many therapies have been advocated, such as chloroform, topical ether, dimethyl sulfoxide (DMSO), and a variety of salves and ointments. These methods have been widely recommended at times, but they have all been proven to be ineffective.

At one time there was also much interest in photodynamic inactivation of the virus after coating the lesions with neutral red dye. However, this initial optimism has been replaced with the fear that this treatment may be carcinogenic. But although there is still no cure for genital herpes, much can be done to ease both the genital lesions and the emotional fear.

I advise patients with genital herpes to keep the area affected clean and dry. I don't believe anyone has invented a better way than the use of soap and water. But be sure to use a nonperfumed soap that doesn't contain deodorants or other potentially irritating chemicals. Some physicians have reported a good response to the use of surgical detergents such as povidone-iodine (betadine). I have also found this to be helpful in some cases, but I always try soap and water first.

It's important to dry the lesions thoroughly after cleansing. Gently patting the area with a towel can be effective, but a hand-held hair dryer does the job without any friction or irritation to the lesions. Take care to avoid overheating the skin.

Remember that heat is irritating to these lesions. So try to keep the area as cool as possible. Shy away from tight-fitting clothing. And avoid activities that increase body temperature, such as athletic participation and sexual intercourse.

Sometimes cool compresses ease the irritation. And if there is a great deal of inflammation and fever, aspirins can be helpful for a short period of time.

Acylovir ointment is the newest drug to treat genital herpes. It is applied to the infected area six times a day for up to 10 days. It may help to lesson the pain of the initial attack and to promote healing. There's also some evidence that it aids in blocking the excretion of the virus. But it does not prevent transmission of the disease, and it has no effect on the course of subsequent lesions. Nor can the drug be used during pregnancy or by nursing mothers.

General hygenic measures must be scrupulously adhered to during an attack of genital herpes. Try to avoid scratching and rubbing the sores. This will help to prevent secondary bacterial infection and the spread of the virus to other parts of the body. Be sure to wash the hands often and never touch the sores and then rub your eyes. And don't expose others to the infection by indulging in sexual intercourse.

Treating the mind is as vital as therapy for the lesions. Too many patients consider themselves social lepers and worry about infecting their partners. But recent studies show there is a practical way to get around this problem.

Dr. James McMahon is an electron microscopist at the Cleveland Clinic. He recently showed that condoms, either the latex type or membrane condoms, are effective barriers to the herpes virus.

The standard industry test for condoms is to fill them with water and place them on blotting paper to see if they leak. But Dr. McMahon examined condoms under the electron microscope when they were magnified 200,000 times. This failed to show any area through which the virus could penetrate.

Remember that the herpes virus is shed for several days after the disappearance of the symptoms and the lesions. Men should therefore use condoms for about two weeks after the disease has faded away. And if you must have intercourse while lesions are present, it's mandatory that condoms be used at that time.

Sex During Pregnancy: Is It Risky?

Is sexual intercourse safe during pregnancy? Several worried readers have written asking this question, wondering if complete abstinence was necessary. Their anxiety was triggered by an article published in the *New England Journal of Medicine*. But does this scientific study give couples sound and practical advice? Or is it causing a needless wave of pregnancy frigidity?

The medical study suggested that women who have intercourse during pregnancy are more likely to develop infection of the amniotic membrane surrounding the fetus. Infections become increasingly frequent if intercourse occurs in the final two weeks of pregnancy. But there was some good news. Whether a couple had intercourse once, twice, or more often a week had no significant effect on the number of infections.

It's an established fact that infection of the amniotic fluid surrounding the fetus is a serious problem. Today it's the single most common cause of intra-uterine death of babies in Canada and the U.S. Last year it was the primary factor in 17 percent of the infants who succumbed.

The result also showed that newborn infants were two to three times more likely to die if the mother had engaged in sexual intercourse. Some deaths occurred because infection was complicated by pneumonia or septicemia. Others failed to survive because inflammation stimulated early labor and the birth of small infants.

It is not known for certain why sexual intercourse has an adverse effect on infant survival. The author of the report suggests that the mobile sperm may carry infection to the amniotic membrane. Or possibly proteolytic enzymes in the male semen help bacteria penetrate the natural barrier protecting the fetus.

During the last weeks of pregnancy risk of infection increases. The rigid cervical opening into the uterus softens at this time, becomes shorter, and dilates. This exposes the area to potential trouble.

How should couples react to these findings? Should they avoid the double bed, move into separate bedrooms, or resort to cold showers for nine months? My initial thought on seeing the headline was similar to one reader. She asked, "Isn't this a rather heavy trip to lay on a couple?"

I don't know the age of the researcher. But he's forgotten what it was like to be young. I doubt that many young husbands will bundle up their sex lives with a big yellow ribbon for nine months. So although the study is of some scientific interest, it contains very little in practical advice. And while reading the original report I could think of ten thousand other unsolved medical problems that would be more productive to investigate.

Reports of this kind also flash a red light in my head. They are basically statistical studies, and their publication in mass media prompts me to repeat an old adage. "There are three kinds of lies: lies, damned lies, and statistics." Even a statistical report dealing with the nation's migraine headaches would arouse my suspicions. But how can you obtain objective truths from 26,000 couples about their sex lives? I think most competent statisticians would use such figures to light the evening fire.

There's another point that concerned couples should keep in mind. Maybe all these figures point to another more logical conclusion. People who approach sex during pregnancy with caution also use this same common sense in other matters. Possibly their newborns fare better because the mother refused to gain 50 pounds during pregnancy. Or managed self-control over alcohol for nine months. Or decided to throw away cigarettes.

The author touches lightly on this fact in the report. For instance, he mentions that blacks have intercourse during pregnancy more than whites. This resulted in a greater number of deaths among black newborns. But was it a greater sex drive that caused the deaths? The report admits it might be related to the differences in social and economic status between blacks and whites.

Does the article prompt me to change my advice to expectant parents? Not one bit. The report simply reinforces at least one longstanding medical opinion about sex during pregnancy.

Few sensible physicians recommend cold showers. Luckily there is a near-100 percent safe way to enjoy sex during pregnancy. Both parties must pay attention to personal hygiene. This means a bath or preferably a shower every day. Then, in the last two or three weeks of pregnancy, husbands might start taking that cold shower. Or if a moonlit night overcomes all self-control, the use of condoms helps to decrease the possibility of infecting the amniotic membrane during pregnancy.

Sex and Athletic Performance

How does sex affect physical activity? Should athletes be locked up for days before an important game? Or is it living in the dark ages to tuck players into bed? And how does intercourse affect the rest of us? We can learn from Casey Stengel, former baseball manager of the New York Yankees, and from an opera singer who struck the right note.

The ancient Greeks believed that seminal fluid was the root of all physical strength. If it wasn't preserved prior to a physical contest, the game was lost before it began. Boxing managers have retained this folklore through the ages. They've firmly maintained that sex before a fight was out of the question. The celibate boxer was meaner and tougher.

Dr. J. Dollard of Yale University gave this theory the scientific nod in 1939. He developed the "frustration-aggression theory," speculating that sexual abstinence increases a person's frustration. This in turn induces aggressive behavior, which is then taken out on an opponent.

But in the harsh world of reality it doesn't always work out that way. For instance, the Minnesota Vikings played the Pittsburgh Steelers in Super Bowl

XI. The Vikings were forced to spend the preceding week away from women. The Steelers could come and go as they pleased. The result? Minnesota lost the game 16 to 6.

Today there are still team managers who are convinced that sex before a game affects the scoreboard. Dr. Donald L. Cooper, director of the Oklahoma State University Hospital and physician to the school's Big Eight college football team, disagrees. He says that intercourse has no effect on performance if it is a regular part of the athlete's life. The majority of doctors associated with sport medicine concur. They maintain that sex helps to combat insomnia and stress before a game. And that by eliminating tension there's an improvement in physical performance.

Some athletes like to pull your leg about sexual activity. One football player admitted that sex made him a little tired, but that he played better when this was the case. He said his sinker worked just fine when he was a trifle fatigued. But if he had all his strength the ball wouldn't sink.

But does the ball ever sink too far? Dr. Cooper reminds athletes that it's mandatory to get the proper amount of sleep after sex. A casual one-night stand will probably leave them exhausted, and the scoreboard empty the next day.

N.N. Baranet, a former coach of high-caliber bicyclists, agrees. She says that intercourse the evening prior to an event is not physically demanding. But if an athlete hunts up a partner a couple of hours before a meet, he or she may as well forget about the meet.

The legendary baseball sage, Casey Stengel, always seemed to hit things on the head. He once remarked, "It wasn't the catching that caused the problem for athletes, it was the chasing." And as one astute team physician philosophized, "The problem is not only keeping the lads away from the lasses, but keeping the lasses away from the lads!"

We can learn something from the performance of an opera singer. Dr. Cooper reminds us that athletes are not the only ones to associate intercourse with a good performance. He relates the story of a famous opera singer who could hit a high C better after sex. It finally reached the point where she refused to go on stage until she had had intercourse.

But what about the rest of us? We're obviously not in the same shape as college football stars, boxers, or possibly opera singers. So I have a word of caution. Research reveals that if intercourse lasts longer than 30 minutes, the body's glycogen stores may be depleted. You'll be exhausted the next day. The solution? If you have enough energy left after sex, rush to the kitchen for a big bowl of spaghetti. By morning the glycogen reserves will be back to normal. You'll roar like a lion!

There's a lack of practical data about this subject, so I have another suggestion for research. Keep an eye on your home-town team. What happens when these athletes return home after a long road trip? Is there a temptation to catch up on lost time? The scoreboard after the next game could provide the answer.

Sex After a Heart Attack

Can you die from intercourse following a coronary? Is it safer to throw in the towel and forget about sex? Maybe switch to hooking rugs or learning to play backgammon? Or could sex be helpful to an injured heart?

Some coronary patients never say die. They have to prove they're still Beau Brummell at the first opportunity. Dr. Stuart Klein, professor at the University of Toronto, talked about this fighting spirit at a medical meeting. He said, "With private rooms in some coronary units, it is not rare for patients to have intercourse within hours or days of an attack."

But most patients are less adventuresome. They become depressed after a coronary. Some fear sudden death during intercourse. Others fret about the chance of relapse. Occasionally couples stop having sex because of the wife's apprehension.

Neither of these two extremes makes sense. You should approach sex after a coronary in the same way you would resume other activities. But patients must understand something about the heart.

A bruised heart needs rest, just like a sprained ankle or a broken bone. Overzealousness could prove fatal. If you are 90 this could be a great way to leave the world. But why push your luck if you're younger? Be patient with your heart. With a little rest it will soon need exercise. That's the time to tackle the big seduction.

Patients often ask how much the heart is strained by intercourse. Here's the good news. Patients with heart disease are often given exercise tolerance tests in hospital. Experts say that these tests cause more strain on the heart than sexual activity. Yet these studies rarely cause a death. In one large series there was one fatality in 10,000 tests.

Some patients give up sex because they were already losing interest even before the attack. But others avoid intercourse for illogical reasons. For example, some post-coronary patients experience anginal pain during excessive exercise. Activity increases the heart rate and blood pressure, requiring more oxygen for the heart muscle. If the coronary arteries can't deliver the oxygen, anginal pain occurs. These people may have to give up running. But they soon learn how fast they can walk, without producing the pain.

Patients often fail to use the same logic with sex. Intercourse also requires more oxygen, so one in five post-coronary patients do develop anginal pain. They should simply learn to slow down. The days of hanging from the chandelier are over. But most couples can develop a more conservative technique that stops the discomfort.

The fragile male ego faces a special trap. Sex is 99 percent in the head, and some men return home with a troubled mind. They harbor deep fears about their ability to perform as before. Too much of this apprehension is fertile breeding ground for male impotence.

How should you prepare for sex after a heart attack? First, try the stairs before returning to the marital bed. Most people use the same energy walking up two flights of stairs as they do in intercourse. Gradually build up exercise tolerance this way. How long it takes depends on the individual, but most heart specialists discourage sexual relations for about eight weeks.

Never set a rigid time schedule for the return to sexual activity. Don't say, "Tonight's the night at 11:45 p.m." Spontaneous sex is always more satisfactory either before or after the coronary. But the urge to resume will hopefully occur in the morning when the mind and body are rested.

Go back to sex with an empty stomach. Celebrating the event with a 10-course meal can cause trouble. A full stomach draws oxygen away from the heart and might produce anginal pain.

What can be done if pain occurs during intercourse? Your doctor might suggest a tablet of nitroglycerine taken prior to sexual activity. This drug dilates the coronary arteries and may prevent discomfort.

Shakespeare gave some sound counsel for coronary patients. He advised the use of alcohol to improve sexual function. But don't forget his caution. A small amount helps, but too much impedes the performance.

Sex is a sound tonic for the mind and heart. Get back to it soon, for no one has designed a more pleasurable way to exercise. If no problems existed before the attack, there should be none following. But first be sure to have your own doctor's approval.

Sex and Lung Disease

"Darling, would you mind if we stop, cuddle, have a glass of wine, and start again?" This is hardly normal bedroom conversation. But my crystal ball suggests this request may occur frequently in North American boudoirs in the future. Increasing numbers of people are developing chronic obstructive lung disease (COLD), a breathing problem that will have a dire effect on their sex lives.

COLD (emphysema, chronic bronchitis, asthma) used to be rare diseases. But they are reaching epidemic proportions. For instance, the U.S. Public Health Service reports that emphysema alone disables 1 in every 14 wage earners over the age of 45. It attacks 500,000 new victims every year. Today COLD is sixth on the list of leading killers, and in terms of general illness second only to coronary heart disease.

Dr. Howard Kravetz, director of pulmonary care at the Good Samaritan Medical Center, Phoenix, Arizona, says the typical patient with COLD is over 50 years of age and male. But a distressing trend is developing. He's seeing more women and young people of both sexes with chronic lung disorders.

Patients who have obstructed airways as a result of asthma, or emphysematous lungs that look like they've been blown up with a bicycle pump, are always fighting for oxygen. Some victims grasp for air while just washing or brushing their teeth. Eventually they become fearful of sex, as strenuous activity, and withdraw from it. Having to eliminate this pleasure then increases their depression.

People with COLD sometimes conclude that the shortness of breath is due to heart disease. The resulting tension contributes to impotence in men and a lack of desire in women. Sexual intercourse becomes as elusive and frustrating as for the dog chasing his tail.

There's another hitch. Patients with COLD or other chronic illnesses are seldom seen by physicians as sexual beings. Since embarrassment usually prevents discussion of sexuality, the topic is seldom raised or explored by doctor and patient. Dr. Roland Freedman of the University of Newcastle-Upon-Tyne, England, says this lack of communication on sexual matters is a universal problem. Like North American physicians, British doctors rarely have antennas tuned to the patient's sexual needs.

Often, however, chronically ill patients send a faint, desperate signal for help. Some will say, "You know, Doctor, things haven't been too good at home for several years," or, "I guess at my age it's normal to lose sexual drive." What they're saying is that they have a sexual problem and want to talk about it. But busy doctors don't always get the message.

What should patients do who notice a shortness of breath during sex? Some quick thinking and a hard look at lifestyle is warranted. Ask yourself whether emphysema, chronic bronchitis, or asthma runs in the family. Do you smoke? Have you noticed more shortness of breath in comparison to others? Or in comparison to your own breathing in the past? And when you cough, are you bringing up yellow or green sputum? If you answer yes to any of these questions, consult a doctor.

Remember that the best treatment of emphysema and other similar problems is prevention. It usually takes 20 or 30 years to develop emphysema. This gives sensible people plenty of time to stop killing themselves with cigarettes. Once smoking stops, there's a marked slowing in the progress of COLD.

But suppose you're starting to puff in the boudoir after abusing your lungs for years. Don't avoid the issue when seeing the doctor. One young chronically ill patient kept complaining of blocked ears. Doctors later discovered another kind of blockage. She had been married four years and could not consummate her marriage.

Some patients have doctors who would never ask directly, "How is your sex life?" If that's the case, pluck up enough courage and inform him of this trouble. But if he starts to squirm in his chair, there's only one solution. You need another doctor.

The majority of patients with COLD don't require a sex therapist or psychiatrist. They need a sympathetic ear and sometimes practical advice on sexual technique. Other partners have to realize that a good sexual relationship does not always depend on intercourse.

Remember, too, that we don't often get something for nothing. Some drugs used to treat the symptoms of COLD can cause a loss of libido. Too many pills, like too much alcohol and tobacco, may hinder sexual response.

But my crystal ball continues to forecast a somber picture. It shows that, because of faulty lifestyle, lung cancer in women will surpass breast malignancies by 1985. This means that COLD will also be on the rampage, that people will be reluctant to toss out bad habits. And that interrupting the lovemaking to have a glass of wine, and then starting all over again, will become the North American pattern.

At What Age Does Sex End?

Oliver Goldsmith wrote in 1773, "I love everything that's old, old friends, old times, old manners, old books, old wine." Today, old wine is still a desirable item, but our society is oblivious to elderly people.

For one thing many older people get little or no advice about sex. Sometimes it's due to their early sex training, or rather the lack of it. Many of them were weaned on the fact that baldness was a sign of virility and masturbation made you insane. It's always hard to replace deep-rooted misconceptions with sensible ideas on sex.

Old people face another stumbling block. In a youth-oriented society, the elderly have lost their appeal. It's not too often that any of us take a second look at an elderly person, and not many companies use an old face to try to sell their products on TV.

Being shoved out of society's eye has to leave some psychological scars. Some people retire prematurely to senior citizens' homes. Others decide they are no longer of any use to the business world. Still others jump too hastily out of their mates' beds. On the surface it seems to be the proper thing to do. But like some old cars, the healthy elderly often have many more miles to go along the road.

Older persons should get the facts right about sex and aging before they decide to call it a day. Kinsey, for instance, found that age had no bearing on the appropriate time for termination of sexual activity. He reported that the oldest sexually active person was an 88-year-old man married to a 90-year-old woman!

In another study, a questionnaire was sent to men 65 years of age and older who were listed in *Who's Who in America*. It was found that 70 percent were engaged in sexual activity. Even in the 75- to 92-year group, about 50 percent were still enjoying a satisfactory sex life. Researchers concluded that a continuing sex life was simply related to reasonable health and willing partners. Being shot by a jealous lover at the age of 95 is obviously still a possibility.

Experts on old age also stress that the elderly need and desire contactual relationships. We all pet old dogs, but there's a general tendency among people to shy away from the elderly. It leaves many senior citizens with a feeling of isolation. Frequently their sincere attempts to establish physical contact are misinterpreted by the young.

The old male who reaches out to touch a young nurse is sometimes considered an old fool making a pass. The sick young male who does the same thing may be making a pass, but no one considers him a fool. Not all old males are lecherous, but society has a habit of thinking so when sexual behavior is exhibited.

Does sex have any medicinal value for the elderly? It certainly hasn't done any of my patients any harm, and helps to relieve personal tensions in an increasingly uptight world. Shying away from sex makes no more sense than tossing away your favorite bottle of wine just because you've reached some magic age. Moreover, if you have a sexual problem, be certain to let the doctor know what's wrong.

Physicians tend to be tuned out about sexual problems in the elderly, so women in particular should nudge him in two specific situations. Today, senile vaginitis is still one of the most overlooked problems in gynecology. A lack of the female hormone estrogen results in painful intercourse when the vaginal lining becomes thin and ulcerated. Failure to mention this trouble to the doctor means there is a good chance it will be missed during examination.

Older women who are about to have a pelvic operation should also remind the doctor that they are still active sexually. If this point is not stressed, too much narrowing of the vagina during surgery may cause painful or impossible relations.

15

The Danger of Diagnostic Radiation

It's been said that even the street dog has his lucky days. Good fortune also happened to me while researching a column. I came across a letter from the Radiation Protection Branch of the Ontario Medical Association. Its contents were hard to believe. And it kindled shock, dismay, and anger. The letter revealed a massive cover-up about the dangers of diagnostic x-rays in Ontario. There's every reason to suspect that other provinces and the U.S. are not immune to this hazard.

What did the letter prove? It stated that patients in one hospital may receive 60 times the radiation exposure given to those in another hospital. For example, measured radiation exposures for a barium meal examination varied between 1.6 R (roentgens) and 90 R. For kidney and barium enema studies some exposures exceeded 100 R, and for special procedures the dose could be several hundred roentgens.

The letter continued, "It is clear that many radiologists are not aware that these high exposures exist and this may make the radiological community vulnerable to criticism by the public or by government. This problem has important implications for the practice of radiology in Ontario." That remark might be the understatement of the decade.

How significant are these figures? They are incredibly large doses of ionizing radiation with life-threatening implications. The effects of radiation are cumulative. That means you can only have so many x-rays of the bowel, broken bones, and dental films in a lifetime. Experts say that our lifetime dose shouldn't exceed 50 R. Yet some patients have been receiving twice this amount in a single set of x-rays from faulty machines and inefficient operators.

But there's more bad news. It's a rare person who has just one x-ray ordered by the doctor. Patients often have films taken of the bowel, gallbladder, kidney, and stomach. An efficient machine could expose them to several hundred roentgens. This is reaching near lethal amounts. A dose of 500 R to the total body causes death.

How could this disastrous situation be allowed to happen? Winston Churchill once said, "Never, never assume anything." He was annoyed at himself after the fall of Singapore. The British leader assumed the naval guns protecting the harbor could be turned landward, but when the Japanese attacked from this direction the guns were useless.

Every practicing physician in North America may have joined Churchill's company. We've been trapped by dangerous assumptions: that x-ray equipment must pass stringent regulations; that radiologists wouldn't subject patients to excessive radiation; that technicians have all been trained in the dangers of radiation exposure. And if a problem existed, the government would inform all doctors.

But there's been an awesome silence about this danger. The Ontario Minister of Health hasn't informed physicians that defective x-ray machines are in use, nor has the Medical Association placed a warning on my desk about poorly trained operators, or even stressed the hazards of ordering multiple sets of x-rays.

I'm not the only one who has been stunned by these findings. A letter from a member of the Radiation Protection Branch of the OMA to another member states, "I'm sure your reaction will be the same as mine to the finding that some examinations deliver 50 to 100 roentgens to the patient. It would seem we have enough data to convince the Ministry they have a problem."

But is this a recent problem? My findings show that the Ontario government has been warned about this menace for several years. One letter from the Board of Radiological Technicians dates back to 1968. A more recent letter to the Minister of Health stresses that continual delay in responding to many reports is placing needless risk on the population. It's the same old story: Too much letter writing, too many closed meetings, and not enough action.

Some critics will label this attack as irresponsible journalism by a medical doctor. They will fear that I will instill in a timorous public a fear of all diagnostic x-rays. Yet if regulatory bodies did their jobs this publicity would not be needed.

Doctors must use x-rays to help them align shattered bones, implant heart pacemakers, and diagnose cancer. Patients should never turn their backs on necessary radiation. But there's an incongruous situation in North America. Citizens will vociferously picket nuclear installation sites. Yet these same people will submit themselves and their families to potentially dangerous x-rays without raising the slightest murmur. They've been led to believe that up-to-date technology has made radiation safe.

You might think, "Modern x-ray equipment must pass stringent regulations. The people using x-rays are highly trained. Besides, we're surrounded by controls for much lesser problems. It simply can't happen."

That's what I thought. But I encountered slipshod attitudes all along the line. Too many people have become blasé about the hazards of radiation exposure. They are assuming everything is controlled when this is far from the truth.

For example, most radiologists couldn't tell me how much radiation patients received from even routine examinations of the bowel, gallbladder, or kidneys. Some said, "You might pick up 1 R." Others stated that they knew at one time but had forgotten. Still others replied that the amount changed from year to year. Or there were tables to figure it out. Or why didn't I check with a teaching hospital?

Alarming responses. It's like a surgeon saying he didn't know how much blood was lost during an operation. Their ignorance was doubly inexcusable since they had already received the letter from the Radiation Protection Branch stressing that some patients were receiving 100 R for these procedures. That report should have started the adrenalin flowing in every radiology department in Canada. Our lifetime dose shouldn't exceed 50 R. Moreover, consider the public outcry when workers receive just 5 R in a nuclear accident.

There were other problems. Some radiologists ignore basic precautions during long x-ray studies such as fluoroscopy. Timing devices, like the buzzer on the stove, are used for this procedure. They warn the doctor when enough radiation has been given for the examination. But timing devices break down and are unrepaired. Or the buzzer sounds and the staff ignore it. Occasionally the dial is turned back to zero to allow more time for the procedure. And some radiologists take three times as many pictures as other doctors.

Why are faulty x-ray machines in use? There's an astonishing reason. Radiologists admit they must crank up the radiation dosage on faltering machines to obtain a good picture. Yet the units are checked only every five years. One technician said the machine hadn't been inspected for 12 years. Others stated that you had to call the government to request an inspection. But x-ray machines are like cars. One month after inspection they may start giving patients too much radiation. Unlucky patients may be exposed to this machine for the next five years.

What about dental offices where batteries of x-rays are now standard procedure? There is an alarming apathy and casualness about x-rays. Most dental technicians interviewed pushed the button but had never heard of a roentgen unit that measures radiation. Several dental assistants told me a full set of x-rays gave the same radiation as a week in the Caribbean sun.

Other technicians naively retired behind office walls when operating x-ray machines. This was a useless exercise. The wall contained no lead to protect them from scatter radiation. And one dentist admitted his x-ray unit hadn't been inspected for 22 years.

The Ministry of Health has been well aware of the dangers to the public from radiation. In 1977 the X-ray Standards Committee filed a report expressing concern about the operators of x-ray equipment. Furthermore, the study observed that patients were receiving excessive amounts of ionizing radiation. Some operators incorrectly positioned people for x-ray. Others failed to use the right cones, filters, and diaphragms to decrease radiation dosage. Still others used the wrong exposure and had to do repeat examinations.

Canadians are not the only ones getting excessive radiation. It was found in

New York State that gonads of some people had been exposed to 200 times the amount of needed radiation. Why? Because the operators centered the beam the wrong way. Even in wrist x-rays the beam was often directed at the gonads!

The report concluded, "A code that does not regulate operators applying the radiation is the same as inspecting a motor vehicle without requiring drivers to have a license." Sensible consumers would say "amen" to that statement.

Surely it borders on criminal negligence that some patients have received monstrous doses of radiation. That they will never know it's happened to them. That faulty machines continue to be used. That there hasn't been an all-out effort to alert everyone to the danger. And that we will all face this hazard until there's a rigid, ongoing inspection of x-ray units.

One last sobering thought. If some hospital x-rays are not safe, what about the ones in private offices? And not just dentists offices—too many radiologists, doctors, chiropractors, and patients have developed x-rayitis. It's a potentially dangerous malady, and it's high time that we learned to protect ourselves and our families from needless radiation.

How? First of all, be a little skeptical about a new concept that is becoming routine in dentistry. Many offices insist on taking batteries of x-rays even before the dentist sees the patient. They maintain that these are required to detect decay in difficult locations and that this procedure constitutes sound dental practice.

Others would strongly disagree. For example, a report on radiological protection condemns this approach as one of the largest abuses of x-rays in dentistry. It stressed that films should only be taken when they're likely to provide significant information. I couldn't agree more.

But I was repeatedly given the same sales pitch when I called dental offices for appointments. I was told not to worry about these routine x-rays. After all, a full set of films was "just the same as spending a week in the Caribbean sun." The dentist would see me after they had been examined. And not a single dental assistant asked me when my last set of x-rays had been taken.

Dental personnel who are so blasé about radiation should be working for Sunshine Tours International. Not one could tell me how many MR (milliroentgens) I'd received from these x-rays, or how much radiation I was allowed during my lifetime. Most had never heard of a roentgen unit that measures the amount of radiation. But they all knew it would cost me approximately $30.

Examining x-rays before seeing a patient borders on malpractice, particularly when the dentist is dealing with young people. Parents should refuse to accept this new routine. Visual inspection is adequate for most children's and teenage teeth, and for some older people as well.

A study a few years ago found that the numbers of dental x-rays seemed to be directly related to a person's income. People have simply been sold a bill of goods by the dental profession. I can imagine the hue and cry if physicians insisted on x-rays prior to physical examination. Or ran up a bill of $70 for x-rays and dental hygiene even before facing the patient. Patients should allow the dentist to take selective x-rays, but the taking of full-mouth films is an unconscionable act. No member of my family will again be subjected to it.

Dental x-rays are not without danger. The lens of the eye receives 50 MR from 16 films. The thyroid gland similarly gets about the same amount of scatter radiation. And some highly respected scientists argue that repeated low-dose radiation is hazardous.

The *Journal of the American Medical Association* raised this warning in 1977. It found that x-ray machines in private offices gave patients twice the radiation of hospital units. In 1976 the *Journal of the Canadian Medical Association* focused attention on chiropractic offices. One article stated, "Reliable authorities believe that the 14 x 36 full-trunk x-ray, so beloved by the chiropractor, presents one of the greatest radiation hazards and published figures show that chiropractors subject 90 percent of their patients to this type of exposure."

The chiropractors I questioned were no more knowledgeable than other professionals about radiation doses. Like everyone else, they had forgotten about safe dosages. Most said they knew the figures in college but couldn't remember them now, even though some had graduated within the year!

You have only one choice when faced with such a calamitous situation. You must use every trick to side-step dangerous radiation. Remember that your body will tolerate only so many x-rays in a lifetime. So never say, "Couldn't you take an x-ray doctor?" It doesn't take too much x-rayitis to use up the 50 allowable roentgens.

Don't forget that tincture of time will cure most aches and pains. That antacids should be tried for an upset stomach before x-rays. That you should shy away from x-rays during pregnancy at all costs. That you should insist on lead shielding for the gonads whenever films are taken. That you should take dental x-rays with you if you change dentists. That mobile x-ray units are best avoided. And don't label your doctor old-fashioned if he fails to order x-rays.

Now is a good time to start your own radiation card, keeping track of the number of times you have been exposed. Show it to the doctor before he orders additional x-rays. By expressing concern about radiation you can circumvent some x-rays. Start asking if the x-ray is really needed. And try to find a dentist who is more concerned about radiation than a week in the Caribbean sun.

How can you know whether or not an x-ray should be done? Very simply, you should follow the same approach as doctors do. They never submit to questionable films. Seasoned physicians know when to opt for x-rays and when it's wise to play for time. And there's no doubt where they would go for x-rays. The person on the street can't be as knowledgeable medically as doctors. But there are some common sense guidelines that can steer you in the right direction.

When do doctors run for x-rays? Lets suppose a 60-year-old physician has never suffered from bowel complaints. Then for no apparent reason there's a change in bowel habits. He may have noticed blood in the stool for the first time, or a tendency towards alternating bouts of constipation and diarrhea. You won't have to ask him twice to get an x-ray to rule out the possibility of cancer.

Another doctor may suddenly pass blood in the urine. During the next hour he's been in touch with a urologist. He's also enquiring whether there's an opening for an x-ray the following day. Similarly a physician who coughs up blood, has a chronic cough, or notices a lump will demand speedy x-rays.

A doctor will also expect x-rays for less obvious reasons. For example, if he experiences abdominal pain, persistent nausea, vomiting, and weight loss, he realizes that x-rays are invaluable to help pinpoint the diagnosis. If x-rays are delayed too long, he will switch to another colleague.

But physicians will play for time when it makes sense. Doctors, like others, sometimes overindulge in food and drink. It may result in bloating, discomfort, and indigestion. But they don't rush for x-rays. They realize that there's a 99.9 percent chance the symptoms are due to gastritis. For a week or two they'll take antacids and give their stomachs a rest. Films will be done only if tincture of time and moderation fail to relieve the symptoms.

Doctors also protect their families from defensive x-rays. It's been estimated that in the U.S. about 30 percent of all x-rays are done for fear of future malpractice suits. Physicians want to use every precaution to guarantee that nothing has been overlooked. It's a tremendous waste of money. It adds needless radiation to a person's lifetime dosage. It's the wrong way to practice medicine. And unfortunately too many defensive x-rays are also done in Canada.

A member of a doctor's family is likely to have a sprained ankle strapped and forget about an x-ray. Similarly, a doctor's child won't be subjected to x-rays of the skull unless there's been a serious injury; doctors know that only 1 in every 1,000 skull films done on children ever shows a fracture. So let your doctor know you don't want defensive x-rays taken. But remember that you must not then run him to court if he misses a slight crack.

Where do doctors go for x-rays? Physicians, knowing the frailties of the human body, are among the world's hypochondriacs. So they want quality when dealing with their own health. That's why they think it's madness to have films done in a chiropractor's office. They're almost unanimous in the conviction that x-rays must be done in the local hospital or a private clinic supervised by radiologists.

What about dental x-rays? Most physicians agree to full-mouth films every few years, then selective ones at yearly visits. But I'm sure they would vehemently object to a complete series of x-rays every six months or even once a year.

How else can you prevent needless radiation? Put yourself in the place of the doctor. Imagine what would enter your mind if a patient said, "Can't you take an x-ray doctor?" Immediately you'd know the patient thought that x-rays were the be-all and end-all of medical diagnosis. That it would be difficult to ease anxiety without one. That trying to talk the patient out of x-rays would probably be a futile exercise. And that the patient might seek another doctor who would oblige by ordering them.

My advice is to remove that phrase from your vocabulary. Never urge your doctor to take x-rays or think he's behind the times for not recommending them. It's much wiser to say, "Would you get x-rays, doctor, if you had this problem?"

Some authorities argue that it's the sole responsibility of professionals to decrease the hazards of excessive radiation. I disagree. It's like saying that drunken driving or drug addiction can only be cured by police officers. Besides, some professionals are caught in a vicious cycle. Radiologists, for instance, can't refuse to take x-rays that are ordered by other physicians. Yet it's frustrating for them to expose people to x-rays they know are done primarily to satisfy a patient's whim.

I think an informed patient can be of great help to family doctors and radiologists. After all, if it works for cancer, why shouldn't it be a sound approach for radiation.

How Safe Is Ultrasound?

Ecclesiastes was wrong. There is something new under the sun. It's ultrasound, and it's becoming the in thing for doctors to use this new diagnostic technique. But is this procedure overrated for accuracy? And when ultrasound waves initiate the fall of a row of dominoes, do they also cause damage to fetal or other human tissues?

Boston radiologists recently sounded a cautionary note at a medical meeting in Washington. Dr. Ted Li of the Harvard Medical School said that "many doctors seem to feel, based purely on intuition, that ultrasound should be performed routinely during pregnancy." He thinks that it's time for them to get off the ultrasound bandwagon.

Dr. Li was concerned that ultrasound screening is providing some patients with a false sense of security. For instance, an ultrasound test diagnosed the existence of twins correctly in 100 percent of pregnancy cases. But in one series it failed to detect infants who lacked kidneys, had clubbed feet, or were missing hands and wrists.

The Boston radiologists emphasized that fetal abnormalities are often too small to be seen by ultrasound or are not visible in all stages of the pregnancy. Equally serious was the finding that ultrasound sometimes diagnoses birth abnormalities that are not present. Moreover, the treatment of pregnant patients is rarely changed by ultrasound diagnosis.

How safe, then, is ultrasound? The use of ultrasound has eliminated exposure of the fetus to x-ray radiation. In addition, to this point, no instances have been reported where ultrasound has harmed patients.

Ultrasound bears no relationship to x-rays, which damage tissue because of the ionizing effect on living cells. Instead, it's a wave form of energy transmitted through the tissues by an oscillation or ripple effect, just as if you were knocking over a row of dominoes. But the long-term safety of this wave of energy has not been established.

The biological effect of ultrasound has been studied in animals. Researchers have shown that ultrasound can cause damage to the cells of a rat's liver and produce cataracts in rabbits. Congenital abnormalities have also been produced in chick embryos and mice. But these abnormalities have occurred at rates of ultrasound exceeding those used in human diagnostic procedures.

I think Ecclesiastes might suggest that medical consumers and doctors should be cautious of new things under the sun. They should remember that in the early years of x-rays it soon became apparent that too much radiation damaged tissues, but it has taken many years to realize that even low-dose radiation can have an adverse effect on the body.

The safety of ultrasound has also been tested by scientists working under well-controlled conditions. But this bears little relation to what actually happens in clinical practice. Today there is a variety of ultrasound equipment on the market. There are sector scanners, real-time scanners, B-mode scanners, and continuous Doppler monitoring devices. Data on the intensity of ultrasound emissions are not easily available. Moreover, manufacturers of these instruments are not required to report this information.

The duration of exposure to ultrasound has been proven to be important, but there are no timers on clinical ultrasound scanners. As well, some technicians using the scanners are poorly trained. Recently there's also been a proliferation of ultrasound scanners in private doctors' offices, and some obstetrical patients have reported being scanned at each prenatal visit!

Today obstetrical societies in both Canada and the U.S., the American Institute of Ultrasound and the National Institute of Health in the U.S. have all stated that obstetrical patients should not be subjected to routine ultrasound scanning. But in 1984 it was estimated that about 80 percent of pregnant women were subjected to his procedure.

It's been aptly said that everything's pretty when 'tis new. I hope this remains so in the case of this new diagnostic technique. But when poorly trained technicians are using machines without timing devices and when the intensity of emissions is unknown, I think medical consumers must exercise caution—perhaps even express some reluctance and skepticism.

16

Death With Dignity

"Please, dear Lord, deliver me in my final days from the physician who has graduated *summa cum laude*, one who is dedicated to prolonging my last breath of life. Rather, grant me the services of a veterinarian, who will treat my suffering with the same cool logic he bestows on wounded animals. I beseech thee, Lord, to answer this, my final prayer."

Sensationalism, you might suspect. But this prayer is heartfelt. I've seen too much misery to joke about the last days of life. Today North American medicine has become cruel and inhumane for the dying. What happens to them would never be allowed to happen to animals. And it shouldn't be condoned for humans either. There is only one solution: a veterinarian should be appointed to every hospital staff.

Veterinarians possess a sympathetic quality lacking in many physicians. They use horse sense in the treatment of terminal disease. They know when they are licked, when it is senseless to prolong agony. And they are not bound by moral, ethical, or religious principles in making the final decision.

Every day as I walk through my own hospital and others in Canada, I'm appalled at the sights I see. Temporary pain is one type of misery. But it can and is usually relieved by the proper use of painkillers.

But repeatedly in 25 years of practice I've seen medical personnel ignore the terminally ill. How do you weigh the quantity of suffering of those lying in bed, paralyzed, for months without hope of recovery? Unable to communicate, unable to feed themselves, unable to have a normal bowel movement? Many elderly patients are incontinent of urine. They lie day after day staring at the ceiling, unable even to scratch an itchy nose.

Veterinarians would never condone this existence for an animal. But some doctors and nurses continue to insist that human life under these conditions still has meaning. I fail to understand the theory that humans must be allowed to suffer just because their brain is larger. And I'd prefer in my last days to be treated like the beloved family pet by the sympathetic veterinarian.

One case illustrates the horror facing North Americans who share my view. For two years a loving family I know watched its father dying, inch by inch, in a nursing home. The patient was paralyzed, incontinent, and incoherent for months. Several times the family was called to the bedside when it appeared death was at hand. Yet the heart continued to beat.

Finally the family asked for help to end this senseless suffering. The doctor was called and told this 85-year-old man had been given the best of care for two years. Now both the patient and family were suffering a hopeless ordeal. The time had come when morphine should be administered every four hours to ease the ungodly death of this man. The doctor agreed and ordered the medication.

Several days passed, but the painkiller was not given. The family, initially relieved by the doctor's compliance, finally inquired why. They were told the nursing staff had decided the patient was not in sufficient pain, so the doctor had rescinded the order. Instead, one tablet of Tylenol was given three times a day. A veterinarian would never have cancelled the order. But doctors do not want to find themselves caught in the cross-currents of controversy. Or to be accused of hastening a patient's demise.

No doubt the nursing staff in the facilities for the elderly are dedicated. It is an onerous task caring for an incontinent, paralyzed patient day after day. Thank God there are nurses willing and able to do the job. But their training is incomplete if they believe physical pain is the only kind of misery.

Today we often hear the remark that people have the right to die with dignity. But they are shallow words. People are still denied sufficient painkillers. Thousands, stricken with chronic disease, are left immobilized, staring silently at the ceiling for months and years, waiting for the heart to cease its relentless pounding. Is this what we mean by dying with dignity? And can we truly define it as painless?

Benjamin Whichcote wrote in 1753, in *Moral and Religious Aphorisms*, "It is base and unworthy to live below the dignity of nature." S.T. Coleridge put it another way in 1817 in *Biographia Literaria*: "By dignity I mean absence of ludicrous and debasing associations." But physicians have proven themselves totally incapable of hearing these words. So the task must be handed to someone else.

I've never heard anyone criticize the judgment of a veterinarian for ending the misery of a stricken pet. No one else has this proven track record. So it's time to appoint a veterinarian to every hospital staff. Surely what's good for a beloved animal is also desirable for humans.

Readers continue to send me letters about this issue. Many ask how they can handle a doctor who doesn't know when he's licked. And questions why individual moral, ethical, or religious principles should so often be the criteria for prolonging life at any cost.

Dr. Dwight Harken, an internationally known heart surgeon and a former professor of mine at the Harvard Medical School recently shocked a medical audience in Edmonton, Alberta. Harken estimates that there are 300,000 "human vegetables" just in the chronic care hospitals in the U.S. He charged that many of these patients are kept alive by intravenous and tube feeding. Harken maintained that these people take up badly needed beds and the time of nursing staff, that society has to face the grim fact that we are no longer able to deliver the best care to all.

His solution? It would be more humane to stop intravenous feeding and allow these human vegetables to starve to death. No doubt his approach numbed some listeners. But Dwight Harken is not a cruel, heartless physician. He's a distinguished surgeon and humanist who has devoted his life to developing new techniques in cardiac surgery that help to prolong productive life. But he also knows there is a time to live and a time to die.

North Americans have been programmed for years to believe that total medical care is their God-given right. The deprogramming process must soon begin. In essence it's the old lifeboat scenario. Who do you toss out of the boat before it sinks? The 45-year-old heart attack victim with a wife and children to support? The child with terminal malignancy? The comatose drug addict who has tried to commit suicide a dozen times? Or the human vegetables?

Isn't it time we asked who is primarily responsible for squeezing the last breath from patients? One could argue that theologians should preach more hell and thunder sermons to denounce this distortion of natural life span. Or why don't they organize a national day of prayer to damn this enormous indignity? But they've already tried to reverse present trends. Several religious denominations have stated publicly that human agony should not be prolonged by extraordinary means. Theologians are not the main suspects.

Alas, I'm sad to say, doctors are the major culprits. They ignore theological edicts. They refuse to take the responsibility for cutting off intravenous feeding. They continue to argue that life-and-death decisions could be abused. They fall back on the argument that it's always been their job to save lives and not pull the plug. But these reasons are all cop-outs.

Physicians are simply reluctant to make a decision that is so open to criticism from their peers or nurses or the patient's family. Or that involves the threat of legal action. Unfortunately some physicians have a deficiency of plain common sense. Years ago they should have formed teams of doctors, theologians, and other consultants to screen patients, ensuring that only the hopeless cases are let go.

History shows that ideas come to fruition when the times demand them. The moment of time must soon arrive when the treatment of humans is equal to that of animals.

Music Therapy

How can families give solace to loved ones who are dying? I have pleaded for the increased use of the Brompton Cocktail and the legalization of heroin for terminal cancer patients. But did I forget something else? Is there power and magic in music for those final days? Should families draw on the soothing tones of Perry Como or a Viennese waltz? Or is music simply an annoyance at this time?

There's no doubt that music has a profound effect on the psyche. Consider the mass hysteria that has accompanied Beatles concerts, or the intense pride felt by Canada's hockey team in 1972 when they stood in Moscow's arena listening to our national anthem. Music can elevate one's mood to great heights.

The early Greeks knew that music had mystic powers. Aristotle investigated ways of purging or purifying the emotions by music. Primitive societies used music as a part of the priest-practitioner's ceremonies. Background music has played a role in medicine and religion for centuries.

A recent article in the Canadian Medical Association *Journal* stresses that today's doctors are missing the boat by ignoring the therapy of music. Dr. B. Mount and Susan Munro reported on how they had helped terminal patients by this means at the Royal Victoria Hospital in Montreal. It should make everyone aware that there's more to relieving pain and anxiety than drugs.

How does music work? It soothes the anxieties of the dying patient in various ways. The Montreal study showed that by promoting muscular relaxation and altering the patient's mood, it also changed the person's perception of pain. It was the only way they could break the vicious cycle of chronic pain in many patients.

There is another big plus to therapeutic use of music. Dying is a lonely experience that can stretch over weeks or months. Music helps to reduce loneliness and eliminates the conspiracy of silence that so often surrounds the dying patient. Music, a pleasant diversion in health, becomes equally comforting at the approach of death.

The Royal Victoria Hospital study covered a wide range of patients problems. The great majority had intractable pain. Others suffered from extreme apprehension. For some, withdrawal from life made nursing care difficult.

Researchers discovered that music means different things to patients. A young woman who had been dynamic and outgoing was plagued by overwhelming panic and pain. She had an attentive family who cared for her every need, but neither their presence nor reassurance could ease the anxiety. Finally a music therapist was asked to see the patient. She prepared a tape of musical selections that was designed to induce relaxation. The effect was impressive. In a short time the woman became relaxed and fell into a deep sleep. During the final days she asked repeatedly for the tape to be played.

Another patient, an elderly Russian lady, isolated by a language barrier, had been extremely difficult to handle. Her therapist obtained a recording of music selections sung by a Russian choir. While it was being played, the patient became alert and in French explained to the therapist her early background. Music opened up new channels of communication in the last days before death.

A 19-year-old youth with advanced cancer had pleaded to die rather than suffer any longer. He, too, found some peace in music. During his previous admissions he had only wanted to listen to rock music, but he soon became intolerant of the repetitive beat. His therapist changed the pace and added Bach, Schubert, and Mozart. These composers became his constant companions towards the end. Equally significant, it became possible to stop painkillers completely.

What should families do who face this problem? There's no need in this instance to feel frustration at not being able to administer heroin. No one can prevent the use of music for a loved one. But you'll have to take the initiative, as music therapists are unavailable in 99 percent of Canadian hospitals. It's also unlikely your doctor will suggest it.

Families will have to use a trial-and-error approach in picking the right music. We all have varying tastes and it could be that some music would be worse than none at all. I'm sure that my family wouldn't offer me the flute or a string quartet. They'd probably bring me some Al Jolson records. Or some music from the roaring 20s. Then just as the pearly gate was about to open, they might chance the pace. Rachmaninoff's stirring second Piano Concerto seems more fitting to me for the grand entry.

The W. Gifford-Jones Living Will

"I'm sorry," the nurse had explained, "but we can't let him have ice cream every day." She was referring to a 85-year-old family friend. He had suffered multiple strokes and was totally bedridden. A mechanical hoist was needed to lift him from the bed to the wheelchair, where he slumped listlessly. His speech was incoherent, his brain damaged by repeated cerebral hemorrhages.

The only thing that elicited a response of pleasure was a dish of ice cream. But it was denied. "Why?" I asked.

"The nursing home can't take the risk of contributing to diabetes in the elderly," I was told. "Sometimes our patients return to hospital. If tests show sugar in the blood, we're accused of causing the problem. Now we can't give daily ice cream without a doctor's order."

Letters indicate that young doctors sometimes take the Hippocratic Oath too seriously. One cited the case of a 91-year-old man with terminal cancer. Nurses thought the man's suffering could be eased by simply prescribing morphine, but the young doctor transferred him to hospital for more tests and x-rays. The man died in hospital within a few days after a fruitless, uncomfortable, and inhumane exercise for those final hours.

Letters to this column repeatedly emphasize that a scoop of ice cream is the least problem facing elderly patients. Nurses frequently write to complain that patients with severe cancer pain are inadequately treated with narcotics. Why? Because the doctor is afraid his patient will become addicted to morphine! Even though he is dying!

My pleas to doctors, nursing home administrators, and families is simple. I'm convinced there comes a time in life when the rules of the game change, a time when patients have the right to say, "To hell with a sound lifestyle. I've used that approach and it's given me a healthier, longer life. But now it's time to go to the dogs."

Does it really matter if my 85-year-old friend gets too much ice cream in his last days? That his blood sugar goes wildly out of control? That he slips peacefully into a diabetic coma and dies? I don't think it matters one damn. But what continues to scare me is that there are still people today, laity and medical personnel, who don't agree.

What can concerned people do? There is no 100 percent way of guaranteeing how life will end, but I've prepared the W. Gifford-Jones Living Will. It stipulates how I want my doctors to act; how I want painkillers to be administered in the terminal days of my life; how my family should act if my colleagues refuse to carry out this philosophy.

Please, Dear Lord, Protect Me from "Bio-Ethics Committees"

"Please, dear Lord, deliver me in my final days from a physician who has graduated *summa cum laude*, one who is dedicated to prolonging my last breath of life. Rather, grant me the services of a veterinarian who will treat my suffering with the same cool logic he bestows on wounded animals. I beseech thee Lord, to answer this my final prayer." This plea was part of the W. Gifford-Jones Living Will in 1982. Now I must add an addendum to protect me in my last days from another Frankenstein monster:

"Please, dear Lord, shield me in the end from a bio-ethics committee. (This is a group of moralists, ethicists, theologians, and doctors who will vote on how and when I should die). Make them understand, dear Lord, that my vote is the one that really matters."

Death with dignity is a relative affair. The banker who collapses on Wall Street, or at the corner of King and Bay in Toronto, hasn't much dignity as he or she struggles for life. But this moment of indignity is miniscule compared to what might happen in the hands of the hospital bio-ethics committee.

Today many hospitals are forming such committees. They contend that medicine has become so complex it's the only way to solve the doctor's dilemma when a decision of life or death must be made. In theory it sounds good. But it reminds me of the story that a camel is a horse designed by a committee.

For instance, one member of a bio-ethics committee told me that kidney transplants should be awarded on a first-come, first-serve basis. But this means the local drunk with a badly deteriorated liver might get the kidney if he arrived five minutes before a healthy, productive member of the community, or even before a young child. Another member was quoted in the press shortly before Karen Quinlan's death in June 1985 as saying he believed she was "very much alive," despite the fact that she had been in a coma for 10 years. Would I want this man deciding whether I should live or die?

Bio-ethics committees deserve some credit for developing guidelines for curtailing "extraordinary measures" when there's no chance of cure. They have also laid down a "protocol," specifying when resuscitation should not be used on a hopelessly ill patient whose heart has stopped. But these measures will end just a fraction of terminal suffering. Bio-ethics committees will be hamstrung by indecision when it comes to tackling the very complex situations of prolonged terminal illness.

The true story of death isn't that of the comatose patient with irreversible brain damage attached to a machine. The real tragedy is that of the conscious patient who struggles with death for days, weeks, or months before the torture ends. Doctors, nurses and families often agree over and over again that it will be a godsend when death occurs. All of them would probably have put their dog to sleep long ago.

Critics of euthanasia claim it is immoral to end life's suffering even when senseless. They argue this is playing God. But this is an impractical philosophical cop-out. God has already placed the stamp of death on the victim. An extra dose of morphine is merely giving God a helping hand.

But in 1985 treating the human patient as humanely as animals is still an impossible dream. We take pride in having created a great democracy with equal individual rights. But there is nothing equal or democratic about terminal illness. Historians will eventually cast a jaundiced eye on those of us who refused to stop the needless suffering of the dying.

If medical consumers must now contend with bio-ethics committees shouldn't they have the democratic right to select members of their own choice. I'd rather take my chance with the local cab driver than someone who believes Karen Quinlan was alive during her 10 years in a coma. All I need on my committee are family members and one trusted physician. I wouldn't mind adding a veterinarian in case one of these loses his head.

Long before I need the committee I'd like to set the ground rules. If I'm riddled with lung cancer and gasping for air hour after hour, don't ignore my plea for help. The law doesn't allow you to shoot me. But it does allow adequate medication. I'd pick a doctor who would provide sufficient drugs to make me insensible to this world.

I'd also remind the committee that pain comes in a variety of packages. If I suffer Alzheimer's Disease, with a reduced mentality of a one-year-old and I'm in diapers, end my life at the earliest possible time. This means saying no to penicillin when I get pneumonia.

I'm attaching a copy of this column to my own Living Will. You may wish to do the same. A copy of the W. Gifford-Jones Living Will may be obtained by sending a donation to the W. Gifford-Jones Foundation, P.O. Box 222, Postal Station A, Toronto, Ontario, M5W 1B2. The primary goal of the Foundation is the alleviation of pain for terminal cancer patients.